Good Computer Validation Practices

Common Sense Implementation

Teri Stokes
Ronald C. Branning
Kenneth G. Chapman
Heinrich J. Hambloch
Anthony J. Trill

Interpharm Press, Inc.
Buffalo Grove, IL

NEW BOOK CONCEPTS

Interpharm Press specializes in publishing books related to applied technology and regulatory affairs impacting the biotechnology, chemical, cosmetic, device, diagnostic or drug manufacturing industries. If you have a manuscript in progress, or are planning to write a book that will be applicable to development, medical, regulatory, manufacturing, quality or engineering professionals, please contact our editorial director.

SOCIAL RESPONSIBILITY PROGRAMS

Interpharm Resources Replenishment Program

Interpharm Press is significantly concerned with the worldwide loss of trees, and the impact of such loss on the environment and the availability of new drug sources. Losses to tropical rain forests are particularly remarkable in that only 3% of all possible endangered plant species have been evaluated for their active drug potential.

Interpharm Press commits to replant trees sufficient to replace those destroyed in meeting the paper needs for Interpharm's publications and advertising. Interpharm is actively supporting reforestation programs in Bangladesh, Israel, Kenya and the United States.

Pharmakos-2000

To foster the teaching of pharmaceutical technology, Interpharm Press has initiated its Pharmakos-2000 program. Under this program, one copy of this book is being sent, at no charge, to every College and School of Pharmacy worldwide. The program covers all 504 establishments listed by the Commonwealth Pharmaceutical Association (CPA) and the Federation Internationale Pharmaceutique (FIP).

It is hoped that this book will be a suitable reference resource to faculty and students advancing the theory and practice of pharmaceutical technology.

10 9 8 7 6 5 4 3 2 1

ISBN: 0-935184-55-4

Copyright © 1994 by Interpharm Press, Inc. All rights reserved.

Interpharm Press, Inc.
1358 Busch Parkway
Buffalo Grove, IL 60089, USA

Phone: + 1 + 708 + 459-8480
Fax: + 1 + 708 + 459-6644

Contents

Appendices

Preface

The team of authors for this book has held as its primary goal the sharing of practical experience in the field of computer systems validation for compliance to Good Practice regulations in pharmaceutical manufacturing, laboratory, and clinical research. The concepts and ideas expressed within this book are those of the authors as individual professionals and are not to be taken as the official policies of their employers.

This book is intended to provide a full complement of specific and useful details for the working professional to make the practice of validating computerized systems, both old and new, a doable activity. The definition of "common sense" as used in this book is "native good judgment" or "good sense in practical matters, gained by experience of life." It is the practical view of what has actually been done in the authors' personal experience across many company environments that dictates the topics, discussions, and advice in this book.

Our choice of two authors based in Europe and two based in the United States was a deliberate decision to have a truly multinational base of experience upon which to draw. The inclusion of a U.K. inspector was also deliberate to give a practical regulatory view from a European perspective.

The authors would like to thank their employers for allowing them to share their professional skills in this way—Digital Equipment Corporation, Genetics Institute, Inc., Pfizer Inc., and the UK Medicines Inspectorate. We would also like to thank our spouses for putting up with us during this book project—M. Suzanne Branning, Betty Chapman, Patricia Trill, and Peter Yensen.

Last but not least, we would like to thank Amy Davis, our editor at Interpharm Press, Inc., for her heroic efforts to meet rather unrealistic publishing schedules with our delayed manuscripts. We all hope that this book will provide a practical and useful service to the drug and device industries for the common sense validation of computerized systems in their regulated environments.

Dr. Teri Stokes, Lead Author
International Consultant, Pharmaceutical Business Group
Digital Equipment Corporation
Basel, Switzerland
March 1, 1994

Team of Authors

Ronald C. Branning
Director, Quality Systems
Genetics Institute, Inc.
Andover, MA, USA

Kenneth G. Chapman
Director, Systems & Planning
Corporate Quality
    Assurance Audit
Pfizer Inc.
Groton, CT, USA

Dr. Heinrich Hambloch
European Consultant
Systems Validation
Good Information
    Technology Practices
Hofheim, Germany

Anthony J. Trill
Principal Medicines Inspector
Medicines Control Agency
London, England

1

Computer Validation Projects, Problems, and Solutions: An Introduction

Anthony J. Trill
Principal Medicines Inspector
Medicines Control Agency
London, England

LARGE PROJECTS—CONTROVERSY AND DISASTERS

There have been a number of high profile, costly, and embarrassing computer project disasters around the world in recent years. The problems have affected civil aviation and commercial, public, and financial sectors alike. To quote from a recent magazine article entitled "Out of Control", which exposed many of the concerns:

> Many people see the fault as lying partly in an unholy alliance between ignorant managers, arrogant consultants, ruthless manufacturers, obstinate software suppliers and, often, a rather reluctant end user.

The article went on to quote from parties involved in various disasters. One deputy public affairs manager referred to:

1

serious mismanagement, possible exploitation by sharp contractors, poor project management and an almost total lack of controls.

The author noted that with so many people and egos, plus sensitive and sophisticated machinery involved, the potential for failure was high—and there were plenty of people to blame when things went wrong. (1)

Commenting on another system failure connected with emergency services the article noted:

> the refusal of management to take into account the high risk involved in their requirements. Contractors were chosen on price rather than quality and no references were taken up. There was an atmosphere of distrust, training was incomplete and inconsistent, there was no ownership of the system by the users. Management felt that the implementation of the system would bring changes in attitudes. (2)

In fact, as the article stated, attitudes needed to be changed at the outset and reference was made to UK DTI reports highlighting the key success factors for systems success. The state of readiness of an organisation and its people is paramount.

These various large system project failures illustrate the complexity of real time interactive systems and the difficulties incurred in defining, designing, developing, and successfully implementing them. The financial and commercial penalties resulting from such failures would have been avoided if proper project and quality management methods had been utilised at the outset and a validated system produced.

PHARMACEUTICALS AND DEVICES—QUALITY AND SAFETY ISSUES

In recent years the author has also seen problems with stand-alone or user configurable systems.

- Analytical instruments (e.g., lack of control over software changes on PC-driven spectrophotometers, resulting in suspect analytical data)

- Automated tablet machines (undetected weight control variations resulting in recalls)

- Autoclaves (retrospective work revealed invalid condition testing logic in the control software for the air removal phase, giving reduced cycle lethality from undetected steam valve malfunctions—resulting in product recalls and impounded batches)

- Batch process control integration (software, interface communications, and data corruption problems)

Other problems have been caused by the overriding or bypassing of computer security systems, such as on-line bar-code readers or check-weighers, resulting in recalls and complaints.

In the devices area an enquiry reported in 1993 on the unnecessary suffering and premature deaths associated with a radiotherapy clinic where patients were accidentally underdosed with X-rays in radiotherapy tumour treatment over a period of 10 years. This was said to be due to human error by a physicist who effectively applied a second correction factor for dose—not realising that the system software automatically applied the correction as well.

These examples illustrate some of the product quality and patient risks resulting from weaknesses in computer controlled equipment, reinforcing the need for validated systems, training, and strict configuration management.

COMPUTERIZED SYSTEMS—PEOPLE AND PROCEDURES

In addition to hardware and software, people and procedures constitute very important quality elements in all aspects of the development and operation of computerized systems.

Figure 1.1 shows a diagrammatic representation of the various elements of a computerized system and is based on an early 1980s PMA paper from the Computer Systems Validation Committee (CSVC) of the U.S. Pharmaceutical Manufacturer's Association (PMA) published by Ken Chapman and his colleagues. (3) It is useful when it comes to considering what is meant by the term *validation* because testing can, in fact, apply to at least seven parts of the system, and we must be clear at all times which part we are addressing. The validation of the controlled part of the system fits well with conventional process validation studies—box 6—but the requirements for validating the contents of box 3—the controlling system—have caused some difficulties over the years. It should be stressed that "people" are very much involved in box 5, and we also have them in the controlling system in box 3. The reader may care to reflect on the validation requirements of these unpredictable multitasking intelligent human components of any computer system.

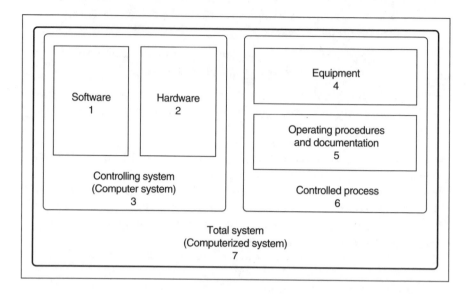

Figure 1.1. Validating a system: differentiation between the controlled and the controlling parts.

This author has found that many of the problems encountered with computer systems are caused by the "people" elements. Many potential users, for example, find it extremely difficult to adequately define the functional requirements or specification for the system; others involved with the development and implementation of the project fail to apply good project management to the various life cycle stages; users/recipients of the delivered system, in the operational and maintenance phase, either do not understand how to use their computer systems properly or fail to comply with the relevant SOPs.

Irrespective of the state of validation documentation, many problems with computer systems are attributable to human beings either not understanding what they are dealing with or not complying with procedures. *The point here is that systems are more than just hardware and software and they are only as reliable as their weakest element.*

BUILDING QUALITY INTO SYSTEMS (SDLC AND GSEP)

Interactive computerized systems are "different" in that simple tests for functional compliance of the final system cannot possibly test the software for all the possible configurations of inputs, processing, and outputs. Rather, strict controls and methods are required over the entire system development life cycle (SDLC) process to ensure that the product from one stage meets its specified requirements before passing on to the next phase. The whole project hinges on an unambiguous functional requirements specification which will be translated through design, coding, testing, system integration, and testing, by an iterative process. At all stages it has to be fully documented and controlled to a QMS and methodology. This is the basis of GSEP (Good Software and Systems Engineering Practices).

Documentation from the SDLC process provides validation evidence of the quality assurance of the *controlling system*. Validation evidence is also required for the *controlled process* (equipment, operating procedures, training of users and support staff, support and control documentation) and ultimately for the *integrated total system* (computerized system).

Inspection

Inspections have revealed system weaknesses, product quality and GMP noncompliances arising from any one or combination of these elements. (4, 5)

Inspectors, not unreasonably, expect to find that controls over computerized systems are at least as good as those applied to noncomputerized systems. Such controls should be reviewed regularly and, where sensible, advance with technological progress as part of the evolution of GMP, GLP, and GCP developments.

EC GMP REQUIREMENTS AND PERSONAL RESPONSIBILITIES

The strengths and weaknesses of computer technology must be taken into account. In the EC, for example, the ultimate responsibility for ensuring that any *systems* (used in manufacturing and quality control) comply with GMP requirements ultimately rests with the people named on the Manufacturing Authorisation (Manufacturing Licence) as legally responsible for Production and Quality Control. This includes the Qualified Person concerned with releasing batches of medicinal products to the market. This responsibility includes knowledge of how well each manufacturing and quality control computerized application is controlled and documented, together with an understanding of potential malfunction risks to data, product, process, and, ultimately, the patient.

EC RULES AND GUIDANCE FOR PHARMACEUTICAL MANUFACTURERS

A recent publication by HMSO for the MCA brings together in one clearly printed volume the texts of the EC Guide to GMP, EC Directives on GMP, The Code of Practice for Qualified Persons and Standard Provisions for Manufacturer's Licences. With its glossy orange cover it may become the new "Orange Guide". (6)

Validation

In the author's view, it is for companies to ensure full validation through comprehensive project management for all new systems projects, so that there is a controlled sequence of events to a SDLC model, fully documented to meet GSEP and GMP requirements. For existing systems impacting on GMP, GLP, and GCP, firms should freeze changes on commencing the project and review their state of compliance with "regulatory" requirements. Where necessary, companies should carry out a risk assessment on such systems to determine validation priorities and develop an appropriate course of action for retrospective work. Salutary lessons were learned by delegates at the recent European Pharmaceutical Technology Conference when they reflected on the figures coming from the case studies, where the costs of "forward" versus "retrospective" validation were quantified as 5 percent compared with at least 30 percent of total project costs respectively, showing the benefits of the life cycle approach to validation. (7)

A mixed state of affairs has been noted in both UK and overseas sites. Systems installed prior to 1989 have generally been poorly documented and controlled. With some older (and some recent) pharmaceutical computerized systems, weaknesses have been noted, such as the following:

- Corporate policies and controls were not developed beyond mainframe business systems. Consistent policies, controls, and system documentation were not in place for PCs, PLCs, and networks used in production or quality control.

- Suppliers had not been audited to ensure that software and systems had been produced in accordance with a system of Quality Assurance (QA).

- No formal contracts had been established covering technical, QA, and GMP requirements for suppliers providing software and systems, and no limits of responsibility were specified.

- Little or no documentation existed for the original system from concept to implementation. (No life cycle validation records or evidence from structural testing).

- There were no system schematics, data flow, or logic diagrams.

- Responsibilities for the system—its documentation, procedures, change control, testing arrangements, and data management—were not defined.

- Design documents drawn up jointly with suppliers were not formally signed off by both parties.

- Qualification and validation arrangements for systems were poor and lacked the following: formal protocols, acceptance criteria, testing procedures, records, reviews, error handling arrangements, formal reporting, and sign-offs.

- Validation test log sheets gave an incomplete record, without explanations.

- Procedures were lacking for controlling changes and no detailed records of changes were kept.

- Detailed written descriptions of the computer systems were not kept up to date.

- No detailed user training records were kept.

- Alarm types and durations were difficult to interpret in process control and environmental monitoring applications.

- Disaster/breakdown arrangements did not work/were not validated. Data was corrupted following power loss and shutdown. Poor recovery, requiring data to be rekeyed on restoration of power.

- Limited storage capacity with overwriting of data on hard disks within several weeks.

- An inability to back up onto diskette or tape drives.

- Original functional design specifications, where existing, did not provide for future extensions or enhancements to the system.

- No routine system audits were performed by QA.

- Noncompliance reports for process or product parameters were lost in a mass of routine acceptable data on piles of printouts (human intervention failure).

- Packaging line security and automation problems (refer to Table 1.1). There have been product quality failures in some instances and batch recalls.

Table 1.1: Security and Automation on Packaging Lines—Design Faults and Misuse

Generally there is far more quality assurance on packaging lines with the various security and automation devices in place. Problems when they do arise are generally caused by human beings. Any one or more of the following reasons may be applicable:

1. Logic and design errors resulting in functional weaknesses for the system (e.g., when a product presence detector is not designed to fail safe). (Often machines with detectors are only engineered to run unless a product fault is detected, no hazard analysis having been undertaken to assess the consequences of detector/sensor failure and whether this would be fail-safe and signal a machine STOP.) Detectors must be engineered to give a positive feedback, during normal running, that everything is OK, and, on failure, signal a machine STOP and alarm/error message.

2. Deliberate changes introduced by human beings during normal running operations by either interfering with, switching off, or overriding on-line security control or monitoring systems (e.g., bar-code reading or check-weighing equipment).

3. Equipment incorrectly set-up and operating out of calibration or limits.

4. Operators simply not following SOPs for the controlled running of the equipment.

Faulty products have reached the market due to the above, resulting in defect reports and batch recalls.

Where there is a resultant risk to pharmaceutical product quality and patient safety, action is required to bring these systems into agreement with the requirements of GMP, GLP, and GCP. It is also important for overseas firms to take note of the EC requirements for such systems if they are intending to export products to the EC.

INFORMATION MANAGEMENT STRATEGIES

Some pharmaceutical firms appear to have Information Systems (IS) departments that are preoccupied with dealing with the maintenance of existing systems or reacting to requests for enhancements.

In such circumstances the author has found that in some firms corporate policies and controls have not developed beyond financial business systems. In such situations, manufacturing and quality control applications, among others, have often been introduced in an uncontrolled and inconsistent manner. However, where firms have clear information management strategies and policies for good business reasons, we find that the quality of integrated manufacturing, quality control, and business systems is of a high order.

CONCLUSIONS

Computerized systems with the potential to affect quality should be clearly defined, documented, and validated. This needs to be done with an appreciation for the different development issues, skills, standards, operational control/security features, and validation requirements necessary for the computerized application.

More attention should also be given to two other major components of computerized systems—people and procedures. These require their own focus for training, competence standards, and validation issues.

International GMP Standards and Inspection criteria also need to be pragmatic, consistent, and harmonized with due recognition being given to the improved process control, data acquisition, and information management that are now possible with these systems.

This author supports the application of logic, common sense, and focused expertise in developing, validating, and managing these systems, in order to avoid "reinventing the wheel" and to contain the workload to sensible proportions dependent on the particular application and risks. His views on such matters can be found in chapter 13.

Other chapters will also provide the "common sense" views of other authors taken from their many years of experience on the industry side, working to ensure good quality, reliable systems in compliance with the requirements of GMP, GLP, and GCP.

REFERENCES

1. Thompson, H. Out of Control. *Intercity Magazine*, p. 31, September 1993. (Available from Redwood Publishing Ltd, 101 Bayham Street, London NW1 0AG.)

2. Ibid., p. 33.

3. PMA/CSVC. Validation Concepts for Computer Systems Used in the Manufacture of Drug Products. *Pharm. Technol.*, 10 (5): 24–34, 1986; and Chapman, K. G. FDA Regulation of Computerized Systems. The MCA Medicines Inspectorate Training Course and Conference, Keele University, April 1989.

4. Tetzlaff, R. F. GMP Documentation Requirements for Automated Systems: Part I. *Pharm. Technol.*, 16 (3): 112–124, March 1992; GMP Documentation Requirements for Automated Systems: Part II. *Pharm. Technol.*, 16 (4): 60–72, April 1992; GMP Documentation Requirements for Automated Systems: Part III, FDA Inspections of Computerized Laboratory Systems. *Pharm. Technol.*, 16 (5): 70–83, May 1992.

5. Trill, A. J. Computerized Systems and GMP—A UK Perspective: Part I: Background, Standards and Methods. *Pharm. Technol. Int.*, 5 (2): 12–26, Feb. 1993; Part II: Inspection Findings. *Pharm. Technol. Int.*, 5 (3): 49–63, Match 1993; Part III: Best Practices and Topical Issues. *Pharm. Technol. Int.*, 5 (5): 17–30, May 1993.

6. Rules and Guidance for Pharmaceutical Manufacturers 1993, MCA, Published by HMSO, PO Box 276, London 5W8 5D7, UK. £11.50 NET (ISBN 0-11-321633-5).

7. First European Pharmaceutical Technology Conference, 13–14 September 1993, Dusseldorf, Conference Proceedings, Advanstar Communications, Advanstar House, Park West, Sealand Road, Chester CH1 4RN, UK.

2

International Regulations and Computer Systems: GCP/GLP/GMP

Dr. Teri Stokes
International Consultant
Pharmaceutical Business Group
Digital Equipment Corporation
Basel, Switzerland

There are some common themes running through the various country regulations for Good Clinical Practice (GCP), Good Laboratory Practice (GLP), and Good Manufacturing Practice (GMP) that have an impact on computer systems and information handling. The challenge for regulated environments is to make sense of these themes and apply them within reasonable limits for the practical needs of the business being conducted. Hence the title of this book—*Good Computer Validation Practices: Common Sense Implementation.*

The European Commission GCP Guidelines became effective in July 1991. Chapter Three (Data Handling) includes some very specific regulatory statements about computer use in clinical trials and remote data entry. This has raised the consciousness of pharmaceutical firms in Europe to a new level of awareness for computer validation. The implementation of ISO 9000 standards for information technology (IT) vendors to the European Communities as of January 1993 further emphasizes the issue of validated quality for information systems and critical software applications.

Section 3.10 of the EC GCP states that "the sponsor must use validated, error-free data processing programs with adequate user documentation." (1) IT professionals are aware that for industry-sized software applications "error-free" programs are still an unrealized goal for today's technology. Therefore, the design of specified validation plans and comprehensive testing protocols is needed to check and validate program performance in GCP and other regulated environments for those systems handling safety, efficacy, and quality data.

This new EC GCP regulatory emphasis brings GCP computer systems into line with the previous focus of many authorities on GLP and GMP computer systems. The UK and Japan have special addenda for their GLP regulations discussing the inspection of computer systems for GLP; the EC published supplementary guidelines for computer systems in Annex 11 of its 1992 GMP. In the United States the Environmental Protection Agency (EPA) has published its Good Automated Laboratory Practices (GALPs) for ensuring data integrity in automated laboratory operations submitting health, environmental, and chemical data to the agency. Computer systems validation has become a global concern for companies operating with regulated environments.

GLP COMPUTER SYSTEMS— UK, JAPAN, UNITED STATES

The United Kingdom—Department of Health

In 1989 the UK Department of Health in London published its GLP Compliance Program for the "Application of GLP Principles to Computer Systems" in laboratories conducting human health and environmental safety studies. The purpose of this compliance program is

> to check that procedures exist to ensure that computer systems are suitably designed, controlled, operated, and maintained in order to properly accommodate the functions and activities to which they are dedicated. The scope of these requirements encompasses any kind of computer system which, in a particular laboratory, is used to capture and/or manipulate raw data in a toxicity or safety study conducted in accordance with the principles of GLP for submission to a regulatory authority. (2)

This UK document continues to interpret the GLP principles for computer systems by including the following five requirements.

1. Identification and Definition of the Systems

   Hardware: manufacture, model, memory size
   Data Storage: disk drives, tape drives, other
   Input/Output: terminals, printers, on-line instruments
   SOPs/Manuals for study systems and subsystems
   Documentation for software and software utilities

2. Control Procedures

   Change control for programs within systems
   Documentation and testing for applications software
   Physical and logical security of systems and software

3. Archives

   Standard operating procedures (SOPs) for raw data storage, archival, and retrieval

4. Quality Assurance

   QA SOPs for monitoring effectiveness of staff and system performance as well as documents, records, and procedures

5. Staff Training

   Documented evidence of qualifications, experience, and training of staff who work with or use the computer system

Japan—The Koseisho

In Japan the Ministry of Health and Welfare (Koseisho) has an attachment to its GLP that details its approach to laboratory computer systems inspections for GLP compliance. It includes many of the same areas of concern as the UK document and looks for similar assurances in SOPs and documented QA practices. The Koseisho gives the following six purposes for such inspections. (3)

1. Computer Hardware and Computer Room

   To check that the host computer is appropriately located in an appropriate condition.

2. Development of Computer System

   To check that the computer system was developed to have an appropriate design and adequate capacity to function.

Software developed in-house. Vendor-supplied systems. Existing system.

3. Operation and Maintenance

   To check that the computer system is operated and maintained to perform the functions as designed.

4. GLP Compliance of the Data Directly Recorded in Computer

   To check that the data processing on the computer system is in compliance with the GLP standard.

5. Computer System Inspection by Quality Assurance Unit (QAU)

   Check that the QAU has inspected the computer system to assure that the system is designed to comply with the GLP standard, developed, and operated to function as designed.

6. In a case where magnetic media of the computer are regarded as raw data, . . . check to confirm that the raw data relating to the study are retrievable.

The United States of America—FDA and EPA

There are two government agencies in the United States that work with Good Laboratory Practices and inspect nonclinical laboratories for compliance: the U.S. Food and Drug Administration (FDA) and the U.S. Environmental Protection Agency (EPA). The position of the FDA is that its 1976 GLP regulations provide enough guidance to support use and inspection of computer systems.

In a 1992 journal article, Paul D. Lepore of the FDA published his view of how the FDA GLP is applied to computerized data acquisition systems. He writes that, "Such systems are considered to be 'equipment' and are regulated similarly to other equipment used in the laboratory." (4)

- Computerized systems are to be of appropriate design and adequate capacity to accomplish protocol directions.

- Their fitness for use in a study is to be documented and monitored by a Quality Assurance Unit.

- Written, approved standard operating procedures (SOPs) are to cover system testing, calibration, standardization, inspection, and maintenance; a historical file is to contain a listing of versions and dates of implementation.

- The system must identify each individual responsible for direct data entry at the time of entry.

- Data entries may be changed but an audit trail must preserve the original entry and identify the person making the change, list the date of the change, and provide a reason for the change.

- FDA's inspections of computerized systems are designed to determine whether the systems operated properly in the past, whether they are currently operating properly, and whether they will continue to operate properly in the future.

The position of the EPA is that the advancement of automated systems technologies in the laboratory call for special guidance in developing documented standard practices to support the EPA GLP requirements. On December 28, 1990, the EPA published a two-part draft document of its Good Automated Laboratory Practices (GALPs) regulations along with an Implementation Guidance Manual. In this document it states the following policy: (5)

It is EPA policy that data collected, analyzed, processed or maintained on automated data collection system(s) in support of health and environmental effects studies be accurate and of sufficient integrity to support effective environmental management. The Good Automated Laboratory Practices (GALPs) ensure the integrity of computer-resident data. They recommend minimum practices and procedures for laboratories that provide data to EPA in support of its health and environmental programs to follow when automating their operations.

This 233-page GALP document is very graphic and user friendly in its approach to helping laboratories understand the GALP regulations as it gives illustrated examples of how each of the regulations could be implemented in the laboratory. Systems people new to the laboratory or laboratory people new to computer systems should find this document a very useful tutorial. It has policy sections and illustrations that cover issues regarding personnel, laboratory management, system responsible person, quality assurance unit, facilities, equipment, security, standard operating procedures, software, data entry, raw data, records and archives, reporting, and comprehensive ongoing testing.

COMMON THEMES—GLP COMPUTER SYSTEMS

A close reading of the documents from all of these country authorities reveals the common themes for GLP computer systems validation to include the following:

- Documented physical and logical security of hardware and software systems, including an inventory of which systems are regulated by GLP.

- Documented installation testing and quality of system design for intended purpose.

- Documented ongoing performance testing of computerized systems to a plan approved and monitored by a Quality Assurance Unit.

- Documented training and experience for staff working with computer systems. This includes GLP training for computer staff.

- Change control SOPs for hardware and software systems and audit trails for data entry changes.

- Documented storage and archiving of raw data that includes testing of the ability to retrieve archived study data.

- SOPs for system operation, data backup, and disaster recovery.

GCP COMPUTER SYSTEMS—SCANDINAVIA, AUSTRALIA, EC, UNITED STATES

The process of conducting clinical trials is highly information intensive. The influence of regulatory requirements for specific documentation at every stage of the process poses a huge burden on the physical handling, reviewing, managing, and storing procedures for documented data within pharmaceutical firms. Computer technology is seen as the only way to effectively address this ever increasing mountain of paperwork for both companies and authorities. The publication of more recent GCP regulations by different countries has reflected their concern for assurance of the integrity of computer resident data in this clinical trial process.

Scandinavia—The Nordic Council on Medicines

The Nordic Guidelines for Good clinical trial practice published in Uppsala in 1989 devotes chapter 8 to Statistics and Data Management. This chapter expresses the basic philosophy that

> The aim of data management is to turn the information from the subject into data in the report, efficiently and without errors. All steps involved in data management should be documented to allow for a step-by-step retrospective assessment of data quality and study performance (audit trail). (6)

Statements specific to computers for other parts of chapter 8 are as follows:

Section 8.2.1 Data Integrity and Transfer

The confidentiality of the database must be secured by procedures with passwords and written assurances by all staff involved. Satisfactory maintenance and back-up procedures for the database must be provided for.

Section 8.2.2 Case Record Form

Basic form design concepts should be followed regardless of protocol. Such concepts relate to consistency in the use of reference codes, terminology and format. Standardization will save time and errors in the design of forms and computer programs used in the data processing and statistical analysis.

Section 8.2.3 Data Quality Assurance

The aim of data quality procedures is to minimize the effects of missing and inaccurate data . . . Data entry should be performed continuously during the course of the study. It should be checked either by double-entry or by proofreading, at least for the primary variables.

Checks for validity and consistency should be on separate items as well as on predetermined combinations of items in the case record forms. Checks should be manual as well as computerized. In the latter case they should, as far as possible, be combined with data entry in order to speed up feedback on data requiring clarification. To supplement the continuous checking of each individual, descriptive statistics on each important variable in the database are useful in the detection of doubtful data.

Section 8.2.4 Code Breaking

When the validation and editing process is concluded, a formal decision to this effect should be recorded. Data for each individual subject should be classified and coded with respect to their inclusion in the various statistical analyses planned to be performed in the study.

After the above actions have been documented, the treatment code can be broken and included in the database for each individual subject.

Chapter 11 of the Nordic Guidelines provides a definition of terms for the document. In this section the definition of raw data includes the following:

> Raw data means all records of original observations or activities in a clinical trial necessary for the reconstruction and evaluation of the trial . . . The term can also include photographic negatives, microfilm or magnetic media. In the case of the latter, dated and verified written transcriptions may replace the originals. (7)

Australia—The Therapeutic Goods Administration

The Australian Therapeutic Goods Administration (TGA) used the Nordic Guidelines heavily as a basis for developing their own Guidelines for Good Clinical Research Practice (GCRP) in Australia, published in December 1991. It also has a chapter 8 devoted to statistics and data management. While most of the statements are similar, there are some more specific computer directions given to certain sections of the GCRP. (8)

8.3.1 Data Integrity and Transfer

The confidentiality of the database must be secured by appropriate standard operating procedures including passwords for all staff involved in the case of a computer database. Satisfactory maintenance and backup procedures for computer databases must be provided.

8.3.3 Data Quality Assurance

The aim of data quality assurance is to minimize the effects of missing and inaccurate data . . . An audit trail should be available to trace the nature of any changes to data, the dates of changes, and the person responsible for the changes.

Data entry should be performed continuously during the course of the study. It should be checked either by double-entry or by proofreading for the primary variables and on a random basis for other parameters.

Checks for validity and consistency of the database should be on separate items as well as on predetermined combinations of items in the CRFs. Checks should be manual as well as computerized. In the latter case they should, as far as possible, be combined with data entry (e.g., immediate automatic checks or batch checking) in order to speed feedback on data requiring clarification.

To supplement the continuous checking of each individual's data during the study, descriptive statistics on each important variable in the database (performed without breaking the code) are useful in the detection of doubtful and/or unusual data.

9.0 Preservation of Records

The documents and any computer records should be retained in a secure place to prevent undue access, loss, or tampering.

9.2 Preservation by the Sponsor

The period for which the documents should be saved is at least 15 years after termination of the study and preferably for the lifetime of the product.

Computer records should be produced in hard copy, which is stored with other paper-based records, to overcome the possibility of loss or inability to read the information due to technological redundancy.

This last statement by the TGA could be read to mean that all computer databases from the trial should be printed out. This would not be practical for many large studies. The commonsense interpretation could be that a company have an SOP to check its archives for retrievability and that if a company is changing computer systems technology, then it must plan for a transfer of its historical clinical trial data on to some other media (possibly, but not necessarily paper) that continues to make that data accessible for audit and inspection.

European Commission—Committee on Proprietary Medicinal Products

The Commission of the European Communities has published its Note for Guidance titled "Good Clinical Practice for Trials on Medicinal Products in the European Community." This was developed by a working party of the Committee on Proprietary Medicinal Products (CPMP) and became effective in July 1991. The objective of this guideline was to establish the GCP standard for trials on medicinal products in human beings within the European Community. It applies to all four phases of clinical investigation of medicinal products.

This document begins with a Glossary of Terms that references computers in the following three items. (9)

1. *Case Report Form (CRF):* a record of the data and other information on each subject in a trial as defined by the protocol. The data may be recorded on any medium, including magnetic and optical carriers, provided that there is assurance of accurate input and presentation, and allows verification.

2. *Documentation:* all records in any form (including documents, magnetic and optical records) describing methods and conduct of the trial, factors affecting the trial and the action taken. These include protocol, copies of submissions and approvals from the authorities and the Ethics Committee, Investigator(s)' curriculum vitae, consent forms, monitor reports, audit certificates, relevant letters, reference ranges, raw data, completed CRF and the Final Report.

3. *Verification/Validation of Data:* the procedure carried out to ensure that the data contained in the final clinical trial report (Final Report) match original observations. These procedures may apply to raw data, hard copy, or electronic CRFs, computer printouts, and statistical analyses and tables.

Essentially the CPMP document acknowledges the current importance of computer technology for data gathering as well as analysis and storage. Chapter 3 (Data Handling) is the most specific about computer use and also references the EEC GMP guidelines for control of computer systems. (10)

Investigator

3.2   Entry to a computerized system is acceptable when controlled as recommended in the EEC guide to GMP.

3.3   If trial data are entered directly into a computer, there must always be adequate safeguard to ensure validation including a signed and dated printout and backup records. Computerized systems should be validated and a detailed description for their use be produced and kept up-to-date.

3.4   All corrections on a CRF and elsewhere in the hard copy raw data must be made in a way that does not obscure the original entry. The correct data must be inserted with the reason for the correction dated and initialed by the investigator. For electronic data processing only authorized persons should be able to enter or modify data in the computer and there should be a record of changes and deletions.

3.5   If data are altered during processing, the alteration must be documented and the system validated.

Sponsor/Monitor

3.10   The sponsor must use validated, error-free data processing programs with adequate user documentation.

3.11   Appropriate measures should be taken by the monitor to avoid overlooking missing data or including logical inconsistencies. If a computer assigns missing values automatically, this should be made clear.

3.12   When electronic data handling systems or remote electronic data entry are employed, SOPs for such systems must be available. Such systems should be designed to allow correction after loading, and the correction must appear in an audit file.

3.13   The sponsor must ensure the greatest possible accuracy when transforming data. It should always be possible to compare the data printout with the original observations and findings.

3.14   The sponsor must be able to identify all data entered pertaining to each subject by means of an unambiguous code.

3.15   If data are transformed during processing, the transformation must be documented and the method validated.

3.16   The sponsor must maintain a list of persons authorized to make corrections and protect access to the data by appropriate security systems.

Archiving of Data

3.17   ... Archived data may be held on microfiche or electronic record, provided that a backup exists and that hard copy can be obtained from it if required.

3.21   All data and documents should be made available if requested by relevant authorities.

The EC GCP document stresses validation, SOPs, adequate user documentation, audit trails, and error-free software programs as important to computer systems that handle clinical trial data. As with the Nordic Council and the TGA, electronic archives must be kept in such a way that hard copy can be retrieved if needed.

The United States of America—FDA

The U.S. FDA provides regulations for GCP, and it has a strong inspection force with legal retribution behind it as a method of enforcing compliance to Good Clinical Practice in human drug trials. There is no single GCP document in the United States as exists in the other countries discussed here. Rather there is a collection of regulations dating back to Tuesday, September 27, 1977, when the FDA published "Clinical Investigations: Proposed Establishment of Regulations on Obligations of Sponsors and Monitors" in the *Federal Register*.

On Tuesday, January 27, 1981, the FDA published a second set of GCP regulations in the *Federal Register*. These were titled "Protection of Human Subjects/Informed Consent/Standards for Institutional Review Boards for Clinical Investigations; and Clinical Investigations Which May Be Reviewed Through Expedited Review Procedure." This document was to clarify existing FDA requirements for informed consent and to provide protection of the rights and welfare of human subjects in research activities under FDA's jurisdiction.

On Thursday, March 19, 1987, the FDA published its 21 CFR Part 312: New Drug Product Regulations; Final Rule. This is commonly known as the IND Rewrite and updates the 1978 regulations. The three sections below refer to retention of and inspection of trial records and reports. (11)

312.58 Inspection of Sponsor's Records and Reports

(a) FDA inspection. A sponsor shall upon request from any properly authorized officer or employee of the Food and Drug Administration, at reasonable times, permit such officer or employee to have access to and copy and verify any records and reports relating to a clinical investigation conducted under this part.

312.62 Investigator Recordkeeping and Record Retention

(a) Disposition of drug. An investigator is required to maintain adequate records of the disposition of the drug, including dates, quantity, and use by subjects.

(b) Case histories. An investigator is required to prepare and maintain adequate and accurate case histories designed to record all observations and other data pertinent to the investigation on each individual treated with the investigational drug or employed as a control in the investigation.

312.68 Inspection of Investigator's Records and Reports

An investigator shall upon request from any properly authorized officer or employee of FDA, at reasonable times, permit such officer or employee to have access to and copy and verify any records or reports made by the investigator pursuant to 312.62. The investigator is not required to divulge subject names unless records of particular individuals require a more detailed study of the cases, or unless there is reason to believe that the records do not represent actual case studies, or do not represent actual results obtained.

None of these FDA GCP documents refers to the use of computerized systems in clinical trials data handling. Does this mean that one can assume that the U.S. FDA does not care about validated systems in clinical trials? Common sense and the FDA's track record of vigorous inspection activity and public debate about validation of computerized systems for GMP suggest otherwise.

Any FDA inspector who wishes to explore the integrity of clinical data held in computerized systems has two FDA working reference documents to use in the investigation of such computer systems.

The Guide to Inspection of Computerized Systems in Drug Processing is commonly known as the "Blue Book" and was published in February 1983. It defines validation as "the assurance, through testing, that hardware or software produces specified and predictable output for any given input." This document discusses inspection strategies for hardware and software validation including worst case limits, multiple testing runs, input/output checks, documentation, backups, and shutdown recovery. (12)

The Technical Reference on Software Development Activities was published in July 1987. It provides reference materials and training aids for investigators and focuses on methods and techniques for the development and management of software. It advocates the Life Cycle approach to building quality into the design of software systems. The preface to this document states the following:

Computer systems are now commonly found controlling activities ranging from the manufacture of animal feeds to the operation of medical device products destined for implant. As these systems become instrumental in assuring the quality, safety, and integrity of FDA regulated products, it becomes extremely important for the Agency to verify that proper controls were employed to assure the correct performance of the computer system prior to its implementation and for the maintenance and monitoring of the system once it has been installed. (13)

COMMON THEMES—GCP COMPUTER SYSTEMS

A review of the GCP documents from these various countries reveals the common themes for GCP computer systems validation to be the following:

- Documented physical and logical security of hardware and software systems.

- Audit trails for data entry changes.

- SOPs for system maintenance and database backups.

- Continuous data entry throughout the trial with validity and consistency checks during entry. These should be both computerized checks and original source document review.

- Documented storage and archiving of raw data that includes maintaining ability to retrieve hard copy of archived data.

- Use of validated, error-free software programs with adequate user documentation.

- Adequate user documentation and SOPs for remote data entry computer systems.

GMP COMPUTER SYSTEMS—PILOT AND PRODUCTION–SPECIFIC GUIDELINES

U.S. FDA Compliance for Computers Under CGMP

In October 1982 the FDA published its first policy guide on computer compliance to Current Good Manufacturing Practices (CGMP). This was CPG 7132a.07, "Computerized Drug Processing; Input/Output Checking." (14) It stated the following:

Input/output checks of data for computer systems, as required by 21 CFR 211.68, are necessary to assure the quality of a drug product processed using such systems. The extent and frequency of input/output checking will be assessed on an individual basis, and should be determined based upon the complexity of the computer system and built in controls.

In December 1982 the FDA published its second policy guide for computer compliance. This was CPG 7132a.08, "Computerized Drug Processing; Identification of 'Persons' on Batch Production and Control Records." (15) This document addressed the need to establish that when a computer checked a process step, it examined the same conditions as a human would look for, and that the degree of computer accuracy in that examination was at least equivalent to human accuracy.

Two months later in February 1983 the FDA published its Blue Book mentioned earlier in this chapter. The Blue Book devoted the whole of its final section to GCMP Guidance. It established the principle that the hardware of a computer system was considered to be "equipment" under CGMP and that all sections of the CGMP regulations relating to equipment would also apply to computer hardware.

In the same final section the Blue Book stated that "In general, software is regarded as records or standard operating procedures (instructions) within the meaning of the CGMP regulations and the corresponding sections of the CGMP regulations apply." (16) It then interpreted eleven examples of such applications.

1. Record Controls. 21 CFR 211.68 (b)

2. Record Access. 21 CFR 211.180 (c)

3. Record Medium. 21 CFR 211.180 (d)

4. Record Retention. 21 CFR 211.180 (a)

5. Computer Programs. FD&C Act. Section 704 (a)

6. Record Review. 21 CFR 211.180 (e)

7. QC Record Review. 21 CFR 211.192

8. Double Check on Computer. 21 CFR 211.101 (d)

9. Documentation. 21 CFR 211.188 (b)(11)

10. Reproduction Accuracy. 21 CFR 211.188 (a)

11. NDA Considerations. 21 CFR 314.8

This original approach to computer system validation under CGMP in the United States produced a flood of conferences, workshops, committee discussions, and white papers. The debate energy expanded beyond the FDA and the pharmaceutical industry to include suppliers of both hardware, software, and integrated application systems. In 1984 and 1985 two further Compliance Policy Guides were published by the FDA. These were CPG 7132a.11, "Computerized Drug Processing; CGMP Applicability to Hardware and Software" (17) and CPG 7132a.12, "Computerized Drug Processing; Vendor Responsibility." (18)

In May 1986 after two years of research, the Computer Systems Validation Committee of the U.S. Pharmaceutical Manufacturers Association (PMA) published its Validation Concepts paper in *Pharmaceutical Technology*. (19) This paper was accepted as a working industry standard for CGMP systems in U.S. drug companies.

The PMA paper defined terminology for computer validation and established the Validation Life Cycle approach. It defined the purpose of a computer system validation program as providing

> documented evidence that a computer has done, is doing, and/or will do, reliably, what it purports to do . . . Computer system validation is a measure taken to ensure that both the hardware and software function as designed and that the process is controlled, or the data processed, as intended. (20)

In April 1987 the FDA published its fifth Compliance Policy Guide CPG 7132a.15, "Computerized Drug Processing; Source Code for Process Control Application Programs." (21) This last CPG raised further discussions among industry, FDA, and suppliers because it recommended that User-firms should do the following:

- Maintain source code for vendor-supplied application programs.

- Review and approve such source code.

- Dead code should be removed on the basis of such reviews.

In December 1987 the PMA Computer Systems Validation Committee (CSVC) once again published a guideline article in *Pharmaceutical Technology* to clarify the key issues listed above. The focus of the article was identified in its title, "Source Code Availability and Vendor-User Relationships." (22) A major contribution of this PMA paper was the definition of four categories of source code.

1. *Operating System:* Utilities, device drivers, compilation tools, etc. No process control functionality.

2a. *Executive:* Instructions for controlling execution of application-specific software.

2b. *Configuration:* Instructions for configuring or compiling application-specific software.

3. *Application-Specific:* Unique to the system instructions that directly reference input and/or output control signals by their logical or symbolic names assigned to them in software.

The PMA stated that "Source code in the application-specific category should be available for routine inspection because it is the most direct manifestation of process-specific operating procedures." (23)

It was becoming clear that the approach established in the FDA's Blue Book of treating computer hardware as "equipment" and software as "records or standard operating procedures (instructions)" did not always fit the evolving characteristics and sophistication of computerized systems used in drug manufacture. In July 1987 the FDA published its Technical Report to educate its inspectors on the activities involved in software development and it referenced the quality standards used in the information technology industry such as ISO 9000 and ANSI/IEEE.

This U.S. FDA/PMA experience with computer system validation under CGMP was widely publicized and formed a background of experience for other countries to use in developing their GMP validation guidelines. Guidelines written in the 1990s have become much more specific about computer recommendations because of the experience base provided by the previous dialogues among the FDA, industry, and systems vendors in the United States in the 1980s.

The European Commission—GMP and Computerized Systems

The Commission of the European Communities adopted two directives laying down principles and guidelines for good manufacturing practice (GMP) for medicinal products in 1991. These principles and guidelines are applicable to all pharmaceutical companies and "are also relevant for all other large scale pharmaceutical manufacturing processes, such as that undertaken in hospitals, for the preparation of products for use in clinical trials." (24)

Annex 11 of the GMP document provides guidelines for the use of computerized systems under GMP and is cross-referenced by the EC GCP. Its contents are stated in full in Appendix D and then compared to the Australian GMP. Other authors in this book also discuss its relevance to their topics of interest, as much of Annex 11 describes a common denominator of good practices (GPs) for computerized systems across all regulated environments.

The chief principle of the EC Annex 11 states that

> Where a computerized system replaces a manual operation, there should be no resultant decrease in product quality or quality assurance. Consideration should be given to the risk of losing aspects of the previous system which could result from reducing the involvement of operators. (25)

The document then continues on with 19 specific recommendations for computer operations in a GMP regulated environment. This is the clearest GMP regulatory document for computers and forms a good basis for developing a quality assurance checklist of computer operational elements to include in validation plans and SOPs in all regulated environments—GCP, GLP, GMP, and CANDA, computer-assisted new drug applications.

The EC GMP Annex 11 states that people should have appropriate training for the management and use of computerized systems within their areas. Appropriate expertise should also be provided for advice on aspects of design, validation, installation, and operation of the computerized system.

Under the EC GMP validation should be considered as part of the life cycle of a computer system. This cycle includes the stages of planning, specification, programming, testing, commissioning, documentation, operation, monitoring, and modifying.

Looking at the rest of Annex 11 for points in common with GLP and GCP needs produces the following list that could serve as a template for a general approach to computer system validation across all three regulated environments. (26)

11.3   Attention should be paid to the siting of the system in suitable conditions where extraneous factors cannot interfere with performance.

11.4   A written detailed description of the system should be produced (including diagrams as appropriate) and kept up to date. It should describe the principles, objectives, security measures, and scope of the system and the main features of the way in which the computer is used and how it interacts with other systems and procedures.

11.5   The software is a critical component of a computerized system. The user of such software should take all reasonable steps to ensure that it has been produced in accordance with a system of Quality Assurance.

11.6   The system should include, where appropriate, built-in checks of the correct entry and processing of data.

11.7   Before a system using a computer is brought into use, it should be thoroughly tested and confirmed as being capable of achieving the desired results. If a manual system is being replaced, the two should be run in parallel for a time, as a part of this testing and validation.

11.8   Data should only be entered or amended by persons authorized to do so. Suitable methods of deterring unauthorized entry of data include the use of keys, pass cards, personal codes, and restricted access to computer terminals. There should be a defined procedure for the issue, cancellation, and alteration of authorization to enter and amend data, including the changing of passwords. Consideration should be given to allowing for recording of attempts to access by unauthorized persons.

11.9   When critical data are being entered manually (for example the weight and batch number of an ingredient during dispensing), an additional check on the accuracy of the record should be made. This check may be done by a second operator or by validated electronic means.

11.10 The system should record the identity of operators entering or confirming critical data. Authority to amend entered data should be restricted to nominated persons. Any alteration to an entry of critical data should be authorized and recorded with the reason for the change. Consideration should be given to building into the system the creation of a complete record or all entries and amendments (an "audit trail").

11.11 Alterations to the system or to a computer program should only be made in accordance with a defined procedure that should include provision for validating, checking, approving, and implementing the change. Such an alteration should be recorded. Every significant modification should be validated.

11.12 For quality auditing purposes, it should be possible to obtain clear printed copies of electronically stored data.

11.13   Data should be secured by physical or electronic means against willful or accidental damage. Stored data should be checked for accessibility, durability, and accuracy. If changes are proposed to the computer equipment or its programs, the above mentioned checks should be performed at a frequency appropriate to the storage medium being used.

11.14   Data should be protected by backing up at regular intervals. Backup data should be stored as long as necessary at a separate and secure location.

11.15   There should be available adequate alternative arrangements for systems that need to be operated in the event of a breakdown. The time required to bring the alternative arrangements into use should be related to the possible urgency of the need to use them.

11.16   The procedures to be followed if the system fails or breaks down should be defined and validated. Any failures and remedial action taken should be recorded.

11.17   A procedure should be established to record and analyze errors and to enable corrective action to be taken.

11.18   When outside agencies are used to provide a computer service, there should be a formal agreement including a clear statement of the responsibilities of that outside agency.

11.19   When the release of batches for sale or supply is carried out using a computerized system, the system should allow for only a Qualified Person to release the batches and it should clearly identify and record the person releasing the batches.

These EC GMP computer guidelines apply to both full production facilities and to clinical trial supplies manufacture wherever they are located and make use of computer automation and control.

Complying with these guidelines should not be seen as just more paperwork for regulatory compliance. From the professional perspective of Information Technology (IT), they provide a structure for maintaining control of the computer environment for more efficient and effective use of computer resources. They also put more structure and control into the human interface to the computer systems. This should provide smoother operation of the computerized business process and better protection for the stored intellectual property of the company.

CONCLUSION

An examination of regulatory documents from many countries shows that there are some common elements for good practices (GPs) with computer systems that transcend the specifics of laboratory, clinic, and/or manufacturing plant. These all have to do with treating the life cycle of computer systems used in regulated environments with as much care and attention to quality as is required for other key "equipment" used in the same regulated areas. The computer is no longer considered a "magic box" apart from the operations it serves.

Validation for Good Practices (GPs) in the data entry process for GLP, GCP, and GMP all involve

- Password security,

- Identification of the entry person,

- An audit trail for data changes, and

- Both logic and consistency checks for related data items.

Both manual and automated checks are recommended by the various authorities.

Other aspects of hardware and software life cycle management have similar common themes across the three regulatory domains. This becomes evident when reviewing EC GMP Annex 11 for Computerized Systems and noting the usefulness of its guidance for addressing GCP and GLP requirements as well as GMP needs.

REFERENCES

1. EC CPMP, *Good Clinical Practice for Trials on Medicinal Products in the European Community* (Brussels: Commission of the European Communities, 1991), p. 23.

2. UK Department of Health, *Good Laboratory Practice United Kingdom Compliance Program: The Application of GLP Principles to Computer Systems* (London: Department of Health, 1989), p. 1.

3. Koseisho, *Good Laboratory Practice Attachment: GLP Inspection of Computer System* (Tokyo: Pharmaceutical Affairs Bureau, Ministry of Health and Welfare, 1988), pp. 157–160.

4. Paul D. Lepore, "FDA's good laboratory practice regulations and computerized data acquisition systems," *Chemometrics and Intelligent Laboratory Systems: Laboratory Information Management*, 1992, Vol. 17, p. 283.

5. U.S. EPA, *Good Automated Laboratory Practices: Recommendations for Ensuring Data Integrity in Automated Laboratory Operations with Implementation Guidance* (Research Triangle Park, NC: U.S. Environmental Protection Agency, 1990), p. 8.

6. Nordic Council, *Good Clinical Trial Practice: Nordic Guidelines* (Uppsala, Sweden: Nordic Council on Medicines, 1989. NLN Publication No. 28), pp. 27–28.

7. Ibid., p. 35.

8. TGA, *Guidelines for Good Clinical Research Practice (GCRP) in Australia* (Woden ACT, Australia: Commonwealth Department of Health, Housing and Community Services, 1991), pp. 28–31.

9. EC CPMP, pp. 4, 5, 9.

10. Ibid., pp. 22–24.

11. FDA, *21 CFR Part 312: New Drug Product Regulations; Final Rule* (Washington, DC: Department of Health and Human Services: *Federal Register*, Thursday, March 19, 1987), Part VII.

12. FDA, *Guide to Inspection of Computerized Systems in Drug Processing* (Washington, DC: U.S. Government Printing Office: 1983-381-166:2001, February 1983).

13. FDA, *Technical Report on Software Development Activities: Reference Materials and Training Aids for Investigators* (Washington, DC: U.S. Government Printing Office, July 1987).

14. FDA, *Compliance Policy Guide No. 7132a.07*, "Computerized Drug Processing; Input/Output Checking." (Available from FDA Freedom of Information Staff (HFI-35), 5600 Fischers Lane, Rockville, MD 20857.)

15. FDA, *Compliance Policy Guide No. 7132a.08*, "Computerized Drug Processing; Identification of 'Persons' on Batch Production and Control Records." (Available from FDA Freedom of Information Staff (HFI-35), 5600 Fischers Lane, Rockville, MD 20857.)

16. FDA, 1983, p. 16.

17. FDA, *Compliance Policy Guide No. 7132a.11*, "Computerized Drug Processing; CGMP Applicability to Hardware and Software." (Available from FDA Freedom of Information Staff (HFI-35), 5600 Fischers Lane, Rockville, MD 20857.)

18. FDA, *Compliance Policy Guide No. 7132a.12*, "Computerized Drug Processing; Vendor Responsibility." (Available from FDA Freedom of Information Staff (HFI-35), 5600 Fischers Lane, Rockville, MD 20857.)

19. PMA, "Validation Concepts for Computer Systems Used in the Manufacture of Drug Products." *Pharmaceutical Technology*. (Eugene, OR: Aster Publishing, May 1986)

20. Ibid.

21. FDA, *Compliance Policy Guide No. 7132a.15*, "Computerized Drug Processing; Source Code for Process Control Application Programs." (Available from FDA Freedom of Information Staff (HFI-35), 5600 Fischers Lane, Rockville, MD 20857.)

22. Chapman, K., "Source Code Availability and Vendor-User Relationships." *Pharmaceutical Technology*. (Eugene, OR: Aster Publishing, December 1987), pp. 24–35.

23. Ibid., p. 32.

24. EC Commission, *Good Manufacturing Practice for Medicinal Products in the European Community* (Brussels: Commission of the European Communities, January 1992), p. 1.

25. Ibid., p. 139.

26. Ibid., pp. 140–142.

3

The Role of Senior Management in Computer Systems Validation

Dr. Teri Stokes
International Consultant
Pharmaceutical Business Group
Digital Equipment Corporation
Basel, Switzerland

As discussed in Chapter 2, U.S. firms have been working with GMP validation of computerized systems for over a decade. This has resulted in a certain visibility for GMP systems validation at the management level. Systems validation for GLP has had a focus in research management, but GCP systems validation remains new territory for all levels of management on a global basis.

In European companies many senior managers find it difficult to consider computer validation as a legitimate topic for their attention and concern. Likewise, many quality assurance (QA) people view computer validation as a specialty task relevant only to computer departments and therefore not a concern to them as they focus on the validation of "mainstream" business processes.

The root of much of this thinking is a fear that one has to know how to program a computer in order to be involved in its validation process. This is an outdated and dangerous way of thinking for the competitive business climate of the 1990s.

Computer networks now operate as the central nervous system of global companies for their activities in research and development, manufacturing, distribution and sales, and finance. Just as the brain contains the intelligence of the individual, the computer systems of a company contain the intellectual capital of the corporation and often control the physical capital as well. Ignoring their existence at strategic levels of the organization is not good business and becomes a high-risk element for industries regulated by government authorities for compliance to GCP, GLP, GMP, and ISO 9000 requirements.

This chapter provides an experience-based approach to help non-computer executives assume their role in computer validation and gain a management perspective of the strategic business needs associated with such validation. Computer experts are welcome to skip this chapter and go on to chapter 4.

WHAT IS THE VALIDATION ROLE OF SENIOR MANAGEMENT?

Taking the pharmaceutical industry as an example, senior management of the company is ultimately responsible to authorities for the safety, efficacy, and quality of company product on the market. Senior management is held responsible for the integrity of data submitted to authorities to prove the safety, efficacy, and quality of company product. Most of that submitted data in today's business environment is resident on company computer systems.

In the case of ISO 9001, the standard clearly describes management responsibilities for systems to assure product quality. It states that

> The supplier's management shall define and document its policy and objectives for, and commitment to, quality. The supplier shall ensure that this policy is understood, implemented, and maintained at all levels in the organization. (1)

This standard also provides a good starting point for senior managers to use in creating a corporate framework for validation of computer systems in regulated environments. Many companies also extend such validation efforts to include mission-critical systems such as payroll and other applications essential to operations, but not directly included in government regulations.

The Role of senior management is to create and enforce a corporate policy document for computer system validation. In the author's experience, the approach shown in Table 3.1 has proven to be practical.

Table 3.1: Corporate Policy Document Approach for Computer System Validation

1. Establish a working group to define company policy and objectives for validation of computer systems in regulated and mission-critical areas.

2. Write a corporate document that states the computer validation policy and quality objectives; include a statement of the company commitment to such policies and objectives.

3. Develop an awareness/education program for delivering this document to all senior managers and to their employees using computerized systems in regulated environments.

4. Prioritize, review, and resource validation projects with funding and work-time to implement the company policy for regulated systems in an orderly way consistent with its statement of corporate quality objectives.

5. Establish a Corporate Computer Validation Advisory Board to monitor and support ongoing validation efforts to meet corporate objectives within company policy guidelines.

All of the activities involved with the Corporate Policy Document approach should be multidisciplinary and involve people from GCP, GLP, GMP, and CANDA user groups as well as QC/QA, regulatory affairs, and data center managers. An objective and independent project manager should drive the document development process.

The project manager's role is to organize working sessions, give a central contact point for collecting all inputs and assuring that project milestones and deadlines are met. An external validation consultant can be used as a resource to provide a broader, noncompany view of validation practices in the industry.

The role of senior management is to sponsor the Corporate Policy Document project and fund it with people and needed resources. The senior group then receives the output document for review and endorsement as official corporate policy. Then management hosts an implementation program to assure its application in all appropriate areas of the company.

Experience has shown that the development of a Corporate Policy Document for computer validation can be done in less than 3 months time if it is implemented as a high priority directive of senior management. Such an activity should be coordinated and driven by a project manager and the work should be done by a team of people who continue in their regular work. Their ongoing daily work using computer applications in regulated environments helps them to keep a reality-based view for developing policies that can actually be implemented within the company's culture and work situation.

Experience has also shown that a clear, concise document of 15–20 pages can cover all aspects of computer validation for corporate level policies and objectives. Adaptation of corporate validation policies to more specific local needs can be developed later at division and department levels. As more detailed directives and standard operating procedures (SOPs) are derived locally, they can still be kept within the framework of the company's Corporate Policy Document and commitment to quality.

WHAT SHOULD A CORPORATE VALIDATION POLICY DOCUMENT CONTAIN?

Each company will have its own priorities for expressing its validation needs in a way that is consistent with its corporate culture and business environment. National companies in Europe will focus more on EC and country-specific regulatory requirements. Global corporations will look to harmonize across the EC, U.S., and Japanese directives.

The topics shown in Table 3.2 are usually covered. It is wise to set the goal of having only one page of text per section topic and to have a consistent format used throughout the document. This makes the document easier to read. The objective of the writing should be the clear and concise communication of corporate policies and validation directives in a way that a noncomputer person can understand. A short list of terms specific to the topic can be defined within each topic discussion for easier understanding by the noncomputer reader.

Table 3.3 shows one format that can be used, having three elements per topic. For each topic there are headings for Management Summary, Definitions List, and Validation Roles/Responsibilities. The Management Summary states in two brief paragraphs what the company policy is for the topic. The Definitions List includes only key terms necessary for understanding the policy issues for that topic. General IT and validation terms would be included in Appendix A. The

Section	Topic
	Table 3.2: Corporate Validation Policies Document: Company XYZ Corporate Policies for Computer Systems Validation
Section	**Topic**
0	Cover letter signed by Executive Committee stating XYZ's commitment to validation policies in the document
1	Business objectives & policies for computer validation
2	Technical objectives & policies for all validated systems
3	Special elements for GCP & CANDA systems validation
4	Special elements for GLP systems validation
5	Special elements for GMP systems validation
6	Role of QA and others in audits and inspections
7	Supplier contracts & audits for internal/external sources of regulated IT products, services, and data
8	Basic elements for validation & testing of computer hardware and networks in regulated environments
9	Validation & testing of computer software and communications interfaces in regulated environments
10	Appendices
	A. IT Terminology, Acronyms, & Definitions
	B. Sample outline of a computer system Validation Plan
	C. Sample outline of a Test Plan for the same system

Validation Roles/Responsibilities heading contains bullet paragraphs (1–3 sentences) of items that need to be addressed in order to implement the policy stated in the Management Summary. The use of bullet paragraphs eliminates the need for transition sentences and extra words. In this way separate ideas can be presented quickly and concisely.

Table 3.3: Example of a Policy Section: Company XYZ Corporate Policies for Computer Systems Validation

---

SECTION 2: Technical objectives & policies for all validated computer systems at XYZ

Management Summary:

This section defines company policy and procedures to be followed when validating computerized systems in regulated environments governed by GXP directives. At XYZ Company, validation shall be considered as part of the complete life cycle of a computerized system. As defined by EC regulation, this life cycle includes the stages of planning, specifying, programming, testing, commissioning, documenting, operating, monitoring, and modifying.

The primary focus of regulatory inspection for computer systems validation is to obtain documented evidence to assure that any system has operated properly in the past, that it is currently operating properly, and that it will continue to operate properly in the future. XYZ policy supports this focus.

Definitions List: (Adapted from ANSI/IEEE Std 729-1983)

Validation Plan: a document written to describe all roles, responsibilities, and activities surrounding the validation of a computer system.

Test Plan: a document prescribing the approach to be taken for intended testing activities under the Validation Plan. The plan typically identifies the items to be tested, the testing to be performed, test schedules, personnel requirements, reporting requirements, evaluation criteria, and any risks requiring contingency planning.

Test Procedure Script: a document written to give detailed instructions for the setup, operation, and evaluation of results for a given test for a specific module of the target system being tested under the Test Plan.

Test Report: a document describing the conduct of and results from testing carried out for a system or system component.

Validation Roles/Responsibilities:

- The functional business manager owning the GXP system is responsible for the validation of a computerized system according to regulatory requirements and must resource the implementation of appropriate validation activities for such a system.

- Appropriate user training shall be documented to show the following:
  —to assure safe and effective use of the computerized system in its validated state
  —to provide methods and procedures for maintaining validation compliance of the system

Continued on next page

Table 3.3 conitinued

* A Validation Plan needs to be developed for GXP regulated software applications and their supporting platform systems. This Validation Plan shall be approved by the System Owner and shall include the following: (Ref: ANSI/IEEE Std 1012-1986)

—Purpose
—Responsibilities
—Reference Documents
—Definitions
—Verification and Validation Overview
—Life Cycle Verification and Validation
—System Verification and Validation Reporting
—Verification and Validation Administrative Procedures

• System validation is to be performed according to the written Validation Plan. This process includes the development of appropriate Standard Operating Procedures (SOPs), Test Plans, testing procedures, specified reports, and so on.

• The System Owner reviews the Validation Report and documents acceptance of the report with a signature and date notation. The System Owner then decides on the continued use or nonuse of the system for regulated environments.

• All documentation from the validation procedure shall be compiled, reviewed, approved, and archived under fireproof and burglarproof conditions. The documentation should also be readily available for audit and inspection purposes.

* Validation documentation must be maintained for the life of the system. If the computer system is classified as a GXP system, the respective GXP archival requirements must be applied.

Management of a GXP System:

• Sufficient change control routines must be maintained and documented for QA and regulatory review of GXP systems.

• Written audit reports shall be reviewed and signed by the functional management owning the GXP system.

• Approved and valid User Manuals shall be available either as paper and/or electronic documents when GXP systems are in use. User Manuals shall be maintained and kept current by the System Responsible Person for the GXP system.

• Appropriate training programs shall be developed, documented, and conducted on an ongoing basis to assure safe and validated use of the GXP system.

• If an electronic signature is to be used in a GXP system, the system must be validated, and system security should be equivalent to or greater than the security in a comparable manual system.

Table 3.3 shows a generic "GXP" set of common requirements for the validation of all regulated systems at XYZ Company. Table 3.4 then references the generic section and discusses only the elements considered to be specific for GLP systems at the company. The work group process of defining the contents for such a corporate document provides a healthy discussion across the regulated disciplines. This results in an awareness of common points of interest and concern that can identify potential risks and foster a sharing of solutions.

HOW DOES ONE IMPLEMENT A CORPORATE VALIDATION POLICY?

Once a company has gone to the effort of developing a specific Corporate Policy Document on systems validation, the next step is adoption and incorporation into company operation. This is often the part that is missing from the project, resulting in the document becoming just another piece of paper gathering dust on a few shelves.

Business managers at division and function level in regulated industries have a history of addressing GCP, GLP, and GMP issues in their operations procedures. Such managers usually, however, have little understanding of the use of computerized systems within those functions. Consequently, they do not consider the manpower needs and resource costs for validating such computer systems.

In many companies computers are still seen as a separate cost item and not integrated among the "real" business issues to be dealt with for strategic/competitive advantage. Not until catastrophe strikes, in such instances as those mentioned by Tony Trill in Chapter 1, do people realize the importance of automated systems and computer-resident data.

In order for validation policies to be implemented within a company, the people controlling the human and financial resource allocations must be made aware of their responsibilities and roles associated with compliance to corporate computer validation policies. The commitment of senior management to this end must be visible to all levels of the corporation. One way to accomplish this is to schedule a series of Validation Policy Awareness events at different levels of the organization. Table 3.5 illustrates this concept.

Table 3.4: Example of a GLP Policy Section: Company XYZ Corporate Policies for Computer Systems Validation

SECTION 4: Special Elements for GLP Systems Validation

Management Summary:

XYZ Company recognizes its responsibility to comply with Good Laboratory Practice (GLP) requirements for validated data in its submission of laboratory results to prove the safety, efficacy, and quality of its products. It is committed to assuring the quality of computerized data systems operating in GLP-regulated environments at all of its facilities. It is also committed to requesting appropriate assurances from contract providers for computer-hosted GLP regulated data.

Definitions List:

GXP/GLP Computerized System: a laboratory computerized system shall be considered operative under this GLP directive if it gathers, stores, analyzes, or reports data for submission to regulatory agencies in support of company claims for the safety, efficacy, or quality of XYZ Company product.

Laboratory Information Management System (LIMS): a software application system that manages data acquisition, analysis, reporting, and workflow within a laboratory.

Validation Roles/Responsibilities:

In general, the standards and guidelines set out in Sections 1 and 2 shall be applied. There are, however, some specific items within the GLP domain that need attention.

* Computer-controlled laboratory instruments operating in a GLP environment shall have the computer element checked and documented for accuracy and proper performance on a regular basis.

* On-line transfer of GLP test results from instruments to a LIMS system shall be verified for accuracy of test data transfer.

* Transmission of GLP data from outside sources shall be verified for accuracy of data transfer. Contracts for such outside services shall require GLP compliance for all data handling activities and systems.

* The Quality Assurance (QA) function shall audit GLP computerized systems on a periodic basis to assure their compliance to GLP validation requirements.

Table 3.5: Implementation Strategy for a Corporate Policy Document on Computer Systems Validation

---

1. Company Executive Committee approves Corporate Policy Document for Computer Systems Validation in Regulated Environments.

2. Division-level Awareness Meeting (hosted by a member of the Executive Committee) reviews the document and establishes decision criteria and a business process for resourcing and prioritizing system validation efforts.

3. Function-level (e.g., production plant or clinical department) Awareness Meeting (hosted by a division-level manager) reviews the document and develops local practices for implementing the policy.

4. System-level Awareness Meeting reviews the document and local practices and identifies a priority system for a validation project. It is hosted by a function-level manager who reviews and approves the Validation Plan, SOPs, Test Plans, and final Validation Report on the chosen system.

5. Each level reports back to its "Host" on a periodic basis describing the progress made or problems encountered in implementing the Corporate Policy Document.

In peer groups at the various management levels, people can review and discuss the Policy Document and examine the practical ways to go about implementing the policies in their own specific areas. Such sessions should begin with a manager, who is senior to the peer group of the session, giving a "kick-off" statement of support for the Corporate Validation Policies.

At the end of the session, the peer group should formulate a discussion summary to go back to that "host" senior manager that explains how they see their way clear to implementing the Validation Policies for their regulated areas. They can also take this opportunity to identify the needed resources to accomplish the implementation.

If there are resource problems, this is one way to identify them up front and give management the opportunity to prioritize validation efforts according to the business strategy of the company. This eliminates the ad hoc approach of most companies where individuals with the interest and budget to validate go ahead and do so on their own with no understanding of the priority to the company for validating their system over other systems.

HOW DO WE GET FROM CORPORATE POLICY TO A VALIDATED SYSTEM?

Part of the corporate document project should include the validation of one strategic system using the new policies. The document working group should identify an appropriate system and serve as a resource to the local system team developing the Validation and Testing Plans. Senior management should fund this effort as a part of the policies project in order to test the workability of those policies in a real situation.

Having accomplished the validation of a system using the Policies, the Appendices to the Policy Document can then include a specific or generic example of the Validation and Test Plans used for this first system. This removes the usual challenge to corporate directives that the plans are too vague to be useful in real situations. It gives the working group tangible proof of their success in developing the Policies Document and accomplishes the validation of a strategic system for the company.

In this way senior management can sponsor, develop, test, approve, and implement workable computer validation policy in a timely and efficient manner. The policy development project also produces tangible results in the validation of one strategic system that can then serve as a reference site for helping others in the company adapt the validation directives to systems in their own areas.

CONCLUSION

Corporate policies for and commitment to computer systems validation for GCP, GLP, and GMP regulated environments must be documented. They must be implemented at all levels of the organization to support the quality standards expressed in ISO 9000. Experience has shown that the methods discussed in this chapter provide a realistic path for senior management to follow in developing and implementing Corporate Computer Validation Policies throughout their organizations.

REFERENCE

1. ISO, *ISO 9001* "International Standard: Quality Systems—Model for quality assurance in design/development, production, installation and servicing" (Geneva, Switzerland: International Organization for Standards, 1987).

4

Documentation Practices and Principles

Kenneth G. Chapman
Director, Systems and Planning
Corporate Quality Assurance Audit
Pfizer Inc.
Groton, CT, USA

This chapter is designed to answer two perennial questions:

1. What documentation is needed for validation projects?

2. How are validation documents best prepared and maintained?

A succinct answer to the first question might be "Only documentation with common sense utility." A corollary applicable to both questions is "the less paperwork, the better."

Unfortunately, many would-be practitioners have been given the false impression that bales of paper represent a primary objective of validation efforts and that acceptability is a function of weight, rather than content.

Most of today's major regulatory agencies are conceptually harmonized with respect to validation of computer-related systems. As can be seen in Appendix D, some regulations, like the EC Annex 11 (1) and Australia's GMP Code (2), are fairly explicit. Others, such as U.S. drug CGMPs (3), are expressed in more general terms. All GMPs, however, describe *what* is to be done, and not *how* to do it; how to do it is generally left to the practitioner, or to various guides and guidelines. The fact that most GMP regulations emphasize the need for documentation probably explains why paperwork is often overdone.

It would be impractical and unproductive to try to list all possible validation documents. Instead, several of the more important ones will be identified and discussed, in order to illustrate why they are needed and how to make them effective.

Every validation document should have an intended purpose, just as every system to be validated has functional requirements. Defining a system's functional requirements is the first and most important step in any validation effort. Similarly, understanding the purpose, or functions, of any validation document before trying to create it will simplify its preparation, optimize its effectiveness, and minimize the paperwork involved.

Table 4.1 identifies nine key documents common to most computer-related system validation projects, with definitions of their functions.

Reasons for documenting validation efforts go beyond simply meeting regulatory needs: They include communicating with regulators, suppliers, employees, management, and the many multidisciplinary principals directly and indirectly concerned with validation and use of the system throughout its life. When the "business" needs for validation documents are effectively met, regulatory requirements, whether GMP-, GLP-, or GCP-related, will also be satisfied.

Before discussing each of the nine key documents listed in Table 4.1, some philosophy, terminology, and general principles are worth reviewing.

VALIDATION DOCUMENT CATEGORIES

In his 1992 three-part series (4), Dr. Tetzlaff postulates that all validation documents can be classified in one of three categories:

1. *Instructions*—documents that define expectations, such as planning documents, protocols, policies, and SOPs.

2. *Events*—documents that record or report events, such as test results, audit observations, and equipment logs.

3. *Reviews*—documents that analyze, evaluate or review, such as data summaries, qualification task reports, investigation reports, and calculated results.

A fourth category is added to include the kind of informational document often needed to support the above:

4. *Information*—documents containing supportive information, such as flowcharts, as-wired diagrams, and glossaries.

Table 4.2 lists examples of documents in each of the above categories.

Table 4.1: Some Key Validation Documents

1. *Company Policies*—state WHAT is to be done.

2. Company, Divisional, Departmental *Standard Operating Procedures* (SOPs)—advise HOW to do it.

3. *Project Validation Plan* (Validation Plan, Master Validation Plan)—describes overall APPROACH (Project-specific).

4. *Functional Requirements*—define WHAT the specific automated System and Subsystems or Modules are intended to DO (often highly iterative: e.g., rapid prototyping).

5. *System Specifications* (Total System Definition, System Design Specifications)—expand on the functional requirements by also embracing physical requirements of the automated system and its operating environment, including all directly related systems and subsystems, whether automated or manual.

6. *Software Quality Assurance Plan*—describes how the structural and functional quality of each category of software will be specifically assured

7. *Qualification Protocols*—experimental plans that describe how Installation Qualification (IQ), Operational Qualification (OQ) and Performance Qualification (PQ) tasks are to be executed. Note that calibration of validation-related, as well as system-related, instruments can straddle all three categories.

8. *Completion Reports* (Task Reports, Project Reports)—describe results of executing qualification protocols and quality assurance plans, usually summarizing the data, results, and conclusions.

9. *Change Control Documents*—describe measures to be taken, or already taken, for restoring validated state-of-control when changes are made to any part of the total system.

Table 4.2: Illustrative Documents by Categories	
Instructions	**Events**
Plans Policies SOPs Master Production & 　Control Records Test Methods Protocols Contract Agreements Functional Requirements Specifications Operating Instructions User Manuals	Batch Records (may also 　include instructions) Test Results Instrument Charts Product Complaints Inventory Records Audit Observations Software Inspection Results Equipment Logs
Reviews	**Information**
Validation Conclusion Reports Qualification Task Reports Data Summaries Calculated Results Investigation Reports Annual Records Reviews Batch Records Reviews Yield of Accountability Yield or Accountability 　Statements	Flowcharts Organization Charts Equipment Diagrams P&ID (piping and 　instrumentation diagrams) As-Built Plans As-Wired Wiring Diagrams I/O (Input/Output) Diagrams Glossaries/Lexicons

DOCUMENT QUALITY

Tetzlaff discusses five elements or attributes he considers important to validation documentation:

1. Written

2. Appropriate

3. Clear

4. Accurate

5. Approved

Three additional attributes are suggested by this author, all of which involve the readers:

6. Available

7. Understood

8. Followed (enforced)

Each of these document characteristics will be briefly addressed from a "common sense" approach.

Written

Handwritten documents, common a century ago, became typewritten documents a few decades ago, and word processor–written today. Most are on paper. Tomorrow's documents appear likely to be written, reviewed, approved, recorded, and distributed electronically.

Regardless of the method or the medium, the purpose of any written document needs to be clearly kept in mind by the author: to communicate (with whom?), to record (why, and for how long?), to comply with regulations (which, and how many?), and so on. In 1979, it was determined by Pfizer's DRUMBEAT™ system (5) that FDA's then-new Drug and Device CGMPs specified more than 130 different kinds of written procedures (SOPs). The purpose of each was defined. Over the next few years, many firms learned it was wise to

*   Generally restrict each SOP to a single subject (less likely to invite "fishing expeditions" by inspectors; easier and more efficient to maintain).

*   Make each SOP available in its current version to all who need it.

*   Follow it.

In computer-related system validation, SOPs often represent components of the system being validated, or of the system's operating environment. Most of the advice that applies to written SOPs also applies to written protocols, records, and other documents involved with validation. A lot of time can be saved and false starts avoided by a well-organized set of practices governing the structure and maintenance of all written documents, whether hard copy or electronic. Tetzlaff describes this as a "procedure for procedures."

Appropriate

A useful measure for minimizing paperwork is to make sure each validation document has a well-defined purpose and that the defined purpose is respected. A common mistake, for example, is to let a functional requirements document declare the type of microprocessor to be used, the number of pixels per screen or the need for a certain operating system. A functional requirements document should define what the system is supposed to do; it directly influences the way new application software will be written or selected and is usually one of the most important of all validation documents. Yet most suppliers and validation practitioners agree that inappropriate advice in the functional requirements document represents the most common, and potentially costly, problem they encounter.

Similarly, it is appropriate for policies and regulations to define what is to be done, for SOPs and guidelines to define how to do it, and for schedules to indicate when it should happen. Mixing such practices usually proves inappropriate and confusing.

Clear

Success of any validation effort depends directly on the clarity and (therefore) effectiveness of communications involved—between project team members, client and consultant, purchaser and supplier, and so on. Measures that help assure clarity resemble those that help assure accuracy:

- Consistent use of standard, well-defined terms (avoid jargon—especially of the "computerese" variety)

- Flowcharts, logic diagrams and other such graphics (the adage is true that "a picture is worth a thousand words")

- Keeping it simple (multisyllable words and flowery language may appear more erudite and sophisticated; but short, simple, clear statements will get the job done more efficiently)

An effective way to assure clarity is to invite editing by an objective (third-party) critic who is not directly involved with the project. The critic should have enough expertise to comprehend the concepts; often, however, the best critic to evaluate clarity is one who will require technical explanations for those portions of marginal clarity.

Defining responsibilities represents an area where clarity is especially important. Superfluous statements, such as "Management is responsible for assuring that this procedure is followed," should be avoided. Explicit statements, such as "The Laboratory Supervisor shall approve the task report to indicate that accuracy of all calculations has been verified," are superior to general statements, like "The Laboratory Supervisor shall sign the task report."

Accurate

Most major validation projects call for voluminous data, beginning at the Installation Qualification stage and continuing through execution of functional test protocols and even into the endless tasks of change control and configuration management. Inaccuracies of such data can cripple a project by requiring nonproductive use of resources to investigate, troubleshoot, and repair.

A fundamental concept recognized by most current validation guidelines and regulations is the need for data entry verification. It is virtually impossible, even for the most conscientious data entry expert, to avoid the occasional transcription error; most individuals will commit several errors per hour of data entry. Yet, once errors are allowed to corrupt a database, locating those errors and correcting them can be tedious, time-consuming, and expensive. Verification measures vary—it is well established that a person cannot find his/her own errors as effectively as can a second party. Often, a database system can be designed to electronically provide "sanity checks"; for instance, required fields that minimize chances for erroneous data entry. Whatever the measure, it is certain that single-entry data will ultimately corrupt the database and must be avoided.

Accuracy is also important in the selection and use of terminology, in defining functional requirements and protocol objectives, and even in spelling and grammatical construction. For a large project, a technical editor is often a worthwhile investment.

Approved

Most validation documents need to be approved—for business reasons and/or for regulatory reasons. The review and approval process can add value, or it can be a time-consuming obstacle to progress.

The number of approval signatures should be minimized; for most documents, two or three should suffice. Each signature should have a defined purpose (e.g., one may be for verifying technical accuracy, another for regulatory and/or corporate policy compliance, etc.).

Documents that contain 10 or 15 approval signatures rarely reflect 10 or 15 thoughtful and responsible approvals. In fact, it has been observed by this author that the quality of a document is often inversely proportional to the number of approval signatures. The reason is that when numerous signatures are called for, their purposes are only vaguely defined at best; each reviewer signs on the assumption that others (who are undoubtedly less busy) have probably done a thorough review job.

Long review periods can de-motivate managers who have been persuaded to write protocols, reports, or procedures. At several points

in the validation life cycle, and especially near the end, when all qualification protocols have been executed, document reviews can sit
squarely on the project's critical path. Measures to accelerate the review
process might include the following:

- Select a strong writer for the initial draft.

- Hold small task group meetings to reach agreement on
  goals and concepts.

- Provide for parallel, rather than sequential, reviews.

- Require review comments crisply within a week or so,
  allowing them to be made informally, in the interest of
  time.

- Have a document manager skilled at resolving differences
  promptly, who calls additional task group meetings, for
  instance, when radical changes are suggested.

Electronic "paperless" review and approval measures can also accelerate the process.

Many documents contain multiple pages, with approval signatures
appearing on the first or last page. To authenticate that the remaining
pages are simultaneously approved, provision is often made for a person to initial each page. Such initialing should occur only *after* the last
approval signature is in place; such practice should be described in a
policy ("SOP for SOPs") and understood by all parties involved.

The *effective date* of the document should be entered only after the
final signature is in place and each continuing page initialed. Word
processing personnel sometimes like to enter the effective date on
a draft, in order to "save time" later on, but this practice suggests to
an inspector that signatures made after the effective date are meaning-
less.

Available

A common mistake is to assume that, so long as a document has been
properly issued, it will be stored for ready retrieval and availability by
all recipients who need it, replaced and updated when appropriate,
and referred to as regularly as necessary. Not true. Not even close in
many instances.

A system should be designed and implemented to assure that each
member of the validation project team has the same information available at all times as other members. This is easily accomplished by carefully planning, organizing, and designing sets of validation manuals

(policy manuals, SOP manuals, operating manuals, etc.). It is important that the manuals are designed for easy and reliable maintenance. Several measures to assure this include

- *Appearance*—notebook binders of professional appearance, personalized with embossed tape, tend to find themselves on top of desks and readily accessible, rather than in drawers or closed file cabinets with their shabbier-looking or anonymous companions.

- *Identification*—especially for larger projects, each manual should be identified by number and location, so that if the holder leaves, the manual can be recalled or reassigned.

- *Organization*—if several sections are involved, section dividers should be used, with a Master Table of Contents in the front of the document to identify all sections. Each section should have its own section table of contents, so that whenever a new document is introduced or one revised, an updated section table of contents can accompany it. This is probably the most effective single measure for assuring reliability of the system, since it enables the manual holder, or any future auditor, to determine quickly if the rest of that section is up-to-date.

Obviously, central control by a document manager, who can periodically inspect the manuals, will benefit most major validation projects.

Understood

Some software suppliers are notorious for the fact that their Operating Manuals are consistently indecipherable. Such suppliers should be avoided or persuaded to take corrective action. There is little purpose served in preparing manuals that cannot be understood.

As mentioned above, use of a third-party critical editor can contribute much to a document's clarity. It is always a good idea to invite several future users of a document to read and criticize it, even taking comprehension tests so the authors can evaluate the effectiveness of communication. A team preparing to execute a qualification protocol can often save itself from false starts or other types of failure by holding a review meeting and discussing exactly what each member plans to do. The many ways that protocols can be misinterpreted can be surprising.

Followed

When the U.S. CGMPs for drugs were finalized in 1979, it was noted they contained requirements for numerous written procedures. Attorneys, as well as FDA officials, at the time advised that

- It was important to have all the procedures specified; and

- It was even more important to ensure that the procedures were being followed.

Similar advice applies to validation documents. If protocols or software development procedures are not followed, all related validation efforts are jeopardized.

Several measures exist to ensure document compliance. The two most common, and probably most effective, are as follows:

1. Personnel training with regard to the specific documents and

2. Auditing, or self-appraising.

The concept of auditing may seem somewhat formal and costly for a validation project, but it need not be either. Instead, a technique of "MBWA" (Management by Walking Around) is recommended. Validation managers can help ensure project success by simply staying in touch with principals responsible for following policies, completing key documents, writing reports, and so on. Informal "auditing" not only helps ensure document compliance, but when done right, reinforces the kind of team attitude that is so vital to validation success.

Formal audits are important for assuring supplier conformance to design specifications and other contractual commitments. Since structural integrity of software depends on how the software is developed, assuring supplier compliance here is often vital. Audit reports should clearly state

- Purpose of the audit

- Observations and conclusions

- Explicit action needed

- How and when such action is expected to be completed

- Status of the supplier, meanwhile (approved, restricted approval, conditional, unapproved, etc.)

Most suppliers are interested in satisfying the customer and will appreciate the advice a professional audit provides; in many cases it helps to make the supplier part of the validation team.

STARTING PRINCIPLES

The objectives of any validation documentation program should be to optimize communications between the writer and all future readers, while minimizing effort needed by all concerned. This requires identifying key potential readers and limiting paperwork wherever possible. Here are some fundamentals that will help achieve the objectives.

Get Organized

Writers and readers benefit when a firm's protocols all follow the same basic format. The same philosophy applies to most other validation documents, such as SOPs, task reports, validation project plans, requests for proposals, and software quality assurance plans. Also, regulatory inspectors can complete their tasks more efficiently (and, probably more enjoyably) if all of a firm's documents within each class follow standard formats.

Mechanical details like pagination, revision numbers, and use of dates are also worth standardizing. All validation documents are developed iteratively (i.e., drafts are prepared, reviewed, revised, reissued, re-reviewed, and finally approved). When validation team members deliberate issues, it helps them to know they are all working with the same draft document, and to be able to refer to specific information by page number or even paragraph number. Today's word processors may be used to automatically date every page, but such capability needs to be used consistently; often, it is worthwhile to provide revision numbers on every page of a document, as well a date.

Consistent use of writing conventions can also facilitate both document readability and change management. Standard terminology, as well as uniform practices involving titles, subtitles, and paragraph formatting, all help the ultimate users of the document; however, this principle can backfire if applied too rigidly—writers need a reasonable level of flexibility.

Another of Tetzlaff's good ideas is the "SOP for SOPs." One well-written policy or SOP that offers guidance on document organization can go a long way in minimizing paperwork.

For moderate- to large-sized validation projects, it is helpful to have a team member serve as documentation coordinator throughout the dynamic phases of the project; with well-organized guidelines in place, this can be an easy task.

Avoid Writing the Same Thing Twice (or More)

As developed in the discussions that follow, the size of most Validation Project Plans can be reduced by having some corporate policies that describe universal validation practices and philosophies of the firm. Similarly, using a single-page supplement to revise a Protocol or Task Report, rather than issuing an entirely revised document, will not only reduce paperwork, but will also help keep the records chronologically consistent.

Use Summaries, Flowcharts, and Tables Effectively

Often, inspectors who request raw data do not really want raw data; they want first-level summaries of the raw data, provided in easily understood tables (some will, of course, insist on seeing raw or original data, which should be maintained in a well-organized manner for efficient retrieval). Likewise, most readers appreciate a concise summary at the beginning of any lengthy document, such as a validation task report; the Task Report Approval Summary, described below, satisfies such a need.

Flowcharts, logic diagrams, decision trees, and other such graphics are useful aids in reducing paperwork and helping readers understand systems and concepts that are being described. Such pictures can be truly worth a thousand words.

Not only do communications within the validation team benefit, but regulatory inspections can also be significantly expedited by a firm's well-organized, well-summarized validation documentation.

Use Prototypes

Once a high-quality document has been created, it can often be used as a prototype, especially with today's available cut-and-paste word processing capabilities. Thus, headers, footers, graphics such as decision trees and logic diagrams, and even text, can be "lifted" from a model document into a new one, and subsequently edited. A model Performance Qualification Protocol, for example, can be cloned repeatedly, saving resources and providing format and convention consistency to generations of new protocols.

Identify the Audience

Each writer should begin with the validation document's most critical potential reader in mind. If the document is a qualification protocol or a task report, that person might be a regulatory inspector. If the document is an operating manual or a system definition, the person should probably be an Application Expert (more commonly known as an "end user"); they are the ones that best understand the true needs of the system, will make the system work, will help get it into a state of control, and will keep it there.

By the way, it should not be assumed that all regulatory inspectors from a given agency will look for the same uniform specification of documents. In fact, such specifications rarely exist. Most inspectors will be favorably persuaded by any well-organized, consistent set of documents based on common sense fundamentals.

Other important audiences might include

- Company officials who will ultimately approve the documents, such as those from quality control, quality assurance, engineering, information technology, regulatory services and the like;

- Suppliers who may need to prepare proposals and specifications that are based on some of the documents; and

- Those who will perform validation work.

By developing a high level of empathy for the reading audience, the writer is more likely to select words and phrases that readers will easily recognize, thereby communicating effectively.

ACTUAL DOCUMENTS

Computer-related validation projects come in all shapes and sizes: the systems may be large or small; new or existing; fully or partially automated; independent or integrated; and so on. Some documents are common to all, such as a software structural integrity statement; most, however, will vary with the nature of each project.

A "small" project might involve one of a dozen microprocessor-driven HPLC (High Performance Liquid Chromatography) units in a laboratory (e.g., where half of the units have already been validated). For such a project, the documentation should be simple, probably matching earlier prototypes in format. Typical contents might include the following:

- List of intended uses (i.e., functional requirements) for the integrated system

- Statement covering acceptability of software structural integrity (discussed below)

- IQ protocol and data sheet for pump, detector, and column; along with system specifications, installation manual, system manual, and as-wired diagrams, if unique
- OQ protocol and data sheet for the pump
- PQ protocol and data sheet for the integrated unit
- Operating Manual

The protocols would be reviewed, approved, and executed; the results analyzed, summarized, and included in a Task Report. All documents would be reviewed and approved according to existing policies. Most documents would probably mimic earlier successful efforts, even photocopies of the starting forms and protocols where appropriate. All documents should be organized efficiently for easy retrieval and reference. Note that all the documents mentioned have business utility.

At the other end of the spectrum might be a large new CIM project involving a fully automated manufacturing operation; an MRP system networked with departments involved in purchasing, materials management, manufacturing, quality control, and financial activities; and a LIMS unit that collects samples and test data, and provides materials status information (release, quarantine, reject) to multiple departments. A project of this magnitude would logically begin with a Validation Project Plan and would probably wind up incorporating many of the documents listed in Table 4.2.

As stated earlier, the nine key documents listed in Table 4.1 will be discussed to illustrate some ways common sense can be applied to all validation-related documentation.

Policies

Depending on size of a firm, its policies may be issued at various levels. In a large, multinational firm, for example, there may be a hierarchy such as the following:

- Corporate (or Company) policies
- Multidivisional Steering Committee policies
- Divisional policies
- Plant policies
- Departmental policies

Obviously, all the above policies should be compatible with each other. Where redundancies exist, consideration should be given to eliminating one or more of the layers. Usually, policies in the aforementioned hierarchy tend to become more detailed as they approach the "front lines," until, at the department level, procedures may be more appropriate.

Validation policies generally describe a firm's philosophy and overall plans. For example, they may define what is to be validated and which organizations are responsible for various aspects, such as supplier interactions, providing design plans, creating and approving protocols and task reports, maintaining records, reviewing contingency and backup plans, auditing and executing the work itself.

Standard Operating Procedures (SOPs)

The SOP is a directive that usually specifies how certain activities are to be accomplished. There are many kinds of SOPs, some of which have different names:

- Manufacturing Instructions
- Standard Test Procedures
- Software Development Procedures
- Security Practices
- Data Entry Procedures
- Equipment Start-up Procedure
- Procedure for Writing Protocols and Task Reports
- Safety Procedures

Since numerous SOPs exist, it is helpful to standardize formats. A reasonable format, for example, might be as follows:

- Purpose (or "Objectives")
- Scope
- Responsibilities
- Highlights (or "Summary," "Synopsis")
- Procedural Steps

In many cases the last category may be unnecessary, since procedural steps could be addressed by the itemized highlights.

Since SOPs are often integral to the system being validated or of its operating environment, accuracy, clarity, and dependable revision control are all essential. Graphics, such as flowcharts, exploded equipment diagrams, and piping or wiring diagrams, can contribute significantly to clarity and understanding.

Validation Project Plan

Tetzlaff, who calls this a "Validation Plan," describes it as a summary document that communicates management's philosophies, expectations, and approaches for establishing performance adequacy. He then outlines its utility for initial top-down and global planning of any medium-to-large validation project. The idea has become popular throughout the industry. The Plan can be used for a single system and its immediate Operating Environment or for a total facility.

The primary purpose of the Validation Project Plan is to identify all systems and subsystems involved in a specific validation effort and the approach by which they will be qualified. Responsibilities and expectations associated with each validation task are normally included.

To keep the Plan wieldy and easy to read, established validation policies and procedures can be referenced, rather than repeated. Similarly, key project-specific documents, such as System Functional Requirements and System Definition, might be identified and possibly abstracted, rather than paraphrased.

Validation Project Plans, as Tetzlaff points out, may assume any number of styles; no single approach is advocated. For a large project multiple Validation Project Plans might be useful (e.g., for LIMS, MRP, electronic batch record system, etc.) with a Master Validation Project Plan to consolidate the overview. Under such circumstances, some centralized document planning and control can contribute significantly to overall consistency and project efficiency. Often, Validation Project Plans tend to evolve even after initial approvals; hence, document maintenance details, including version identification, pagination, and dating each page can be important.

An illustrative table of contents for a Validation Project Plan covering the above LIMS subsystem is provided in Appendix 4.1 of this chapter.

Functional Requirements

The importance of the *functional requirements* definition is often underestimated; yet, this document is the one most likely to affect success of the project. Historically, the terms *functional requirements* and *system specifications* have been frequently combined and confused, with the result that no one knows exactly what the system is supposed to do. One reason for this confusion is that, to adequately define a system's functional requirements a variety of application experts (end users) need to be identified and consulted. This requires empathy and a commitment of resources; but the investment offers great returns.

Defining functional requirements should include maximum input from representative potential end users of the system. Musts and wants should be identified as such, and the wants prioritized.

Figure 4.1 illustrates how several key documents in the Validation Project Plan merge at the start of a new system Development Life Cycle. An important point not illustrated is that all steps following the System Definition are usually iterative, as feedback is obtained from many disciplines and from potential suppliers. This feedback often includes new evolving technology that can be of great value to end users as well as the project planners and might influence the functional requirements, especially in the *Wants* column. On smaller projects, there may not be need for the RFP (Request for Proposal); but the principles and iterative nature of the activities normally still apply.

System Specifications

This document represents the foundation for the validation effort. It describes clearly and completely how the system will operate and how it will satisfy the system's defined *functional requirements*.

System Specifications should provide all the information needed for installation, operational, and performance qualification efforts, addressing both normal and abnormal operating modes. Cross-referencing other documents, such as operating manuals, SOPs, equipment drawings, and flowcharts, is often appropriate; hence, reliable document management and change control measures are essential.

System Specifications can be finalized only after vendors and specific hardware and software have been selected. It often helps to make key vendors part of the team that finalizes the System Specifications and plans the validation effort.

Software Quality Assurance Plan (SQAP)

Assurance of software quality is vital to system validation. Libraries of books have been written on the subject. IEEE/ANSI (6) represents an excellent source of definitions and standards concerning software quality assurance; many definitions in this book originate with that source. However, it must be remembered that IEEE/ANSI focuses primarily on software, whereas this book addresses total systems; thus, some term definitions do not exactly match. A key term not defined by IEEE/ANSI, for example, is the *canned configurable*, which will be discussed here.

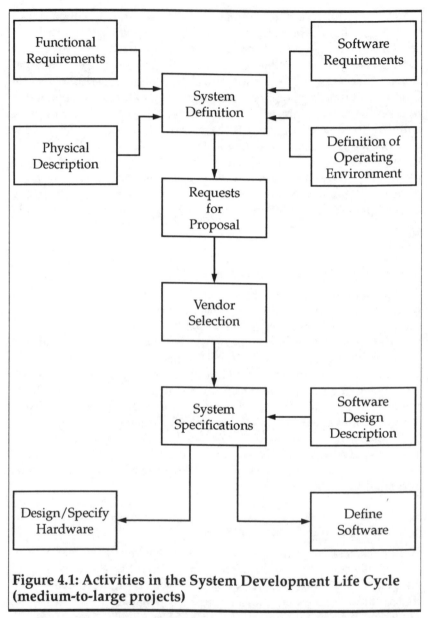

Figure 4.1: Activities in the System Development Life Cycle (medium-to-large projects)

For practical purposes, all forms of software testing can be grouped into two major categories: structural testing and functional testing. Both test methods are important. Structural testing applies only to software, whereas functional testing can be usefully applied to total systems that include software and hardware.

Functional testing is also known as "Blackbox Testing," since it is conducted independently of the source code. Functional testing involves matching actual output against predicted output, based on defined test inputs, all of which are normally expressed in a Functional Test Protocol. The test inputs are usually designed to embrace all important boundary conditions. The Functional Test Protocol requires input from Application Experts (end users), as well as software experts; it is often helpful to include participation by the software and/or hardware supplier, as well.

Structural testing involves the source code and the implementation details. It can include examination of programming standards, style and control methods, source language, database design, and the like. Structural testing can only be conducted by software experts. The best time for structural testing to be conducted is during software development. For that reason, it is important that structural testing be an integral component of software development procedures. The adage that "quality must be built into software; it cannot be tested in" is fundamental, and is especially applicable to structural testing.

An important corollary is that, once structural testing needs have been satisfied (i.e., structural integrity has been verified), validation of a computer-based system can be based on functional testing alone. Recognition of this corollary can significantly simplify the validation planning effort.

IEEE portrays software in two general categories: Application Software and System Software. *Application software* is highly specific to individual user-firm needs. *Systems software*, which includes the operating system, does not directly control functionality of the application software.

A third category that has emerged and now dominates the market is called *configurable software*, which satisfies neither of the above definitions (7). Viewed from the system software, configurable software "looks like" an application program; viewed from the application program, configurable software is a "platform," much like an operating system. If the configurable software is modified or "customized" to a specific user's needs, it becomes an application program by definition and is called a "custom configurable"; when purchased "off the shelf," it is known as a "canned configurable." Lotus 1-2-3™ is a widely recognized example of the *canned configurable*.

Whether the software is developed in-house or purchased, and regardless of its classification, all software is functionally tested as part of the validation program. System software and configurable software are automatically exercised when the application program is functionally tested. Test plans are best developed collaboratively by the software developer and the application expert (end user) and should include testing of all key outer boundary conditions. Both the plan and the results should be documented.

Assurance of structural quality is somewhat more complex, especially for purchased software. In the case of application software or custom configurables, the first step is to assure, usually through auditing, that the vendor has built quality into the software using techniques equivalent to those the user-firm itself would have used. Inspection of vendor SOPs and of the source code by an audit team that includes someone expert in computer science is appropriate. Table 4.3 illustrates a typical software quality assurance checklist.

In the case of operating systems, executive software, or canned configurables, for which auditing may be impractical or even impossible, the corresponding first step is to determine whether the software has gained enough successful experience, in its present version, to warrant the conclusion that its structural testing requirements have been satisfied.

Qualification Protocols

Qualification Protocols are experimental plans that describe how Installation Qualification (IQ), Operational Qualification (OQ) and Performance Qualification (PQ) tasks are to be executed. Careful planning and systematization can significantly help to minimize volume, tedium, and cost of protocols.

For example, use of standard forms can either help or hinder, depending on the flexibility of their design. Some standard forms are so rigidly designed that only a line or two of data are entered per page, which creates excessive amounts of paper. An efficient protocol might identify the key objectives, team principals, action plan summary, other highlights and approval signatures and dates on the cover page. Where practical, references should be made to other documents that are relevant to the experiment, rather than including copies as part of the protocol. Checklist items are useful to verify that all validation-related instruments are in a state of calibration and any applicable safety instructions are prominently displayed. Stepwise experimental instructions then usually constitute the balance of the protocol.

Protocol change control practices present opportunities for significant paper reduction. Often, evidence gathered during initial experimental efforts reveals the need to alter the protocol, either because of new information or the discovery of prior oversights. Rather than rewrite the protocol, which is not only costly but also complicates the

Table 4.3: Software Vendor Audit Checklist

1.0　General Company Information

　　1.01　History
　　1.02　Size
　　1.03　Financial Background
　　1.04　Future
　　1.05　Separate and Independent QC unit
　　1.06　Knowledge of Contemporary Computer Validation
　　　　　Practices Within the Pharmaceutical Industry
　　1.07　Programmers' Qualifications

2.0　Documents (SOPs) Defining Programming Standards

3.0　Documents (SOPs) Defining Software Development Practices

4.0　Documents (SOPs) Defining Structural and Functional Testing
　　　and Recording of Test Results

5.0　Software Quality Assurance Program

6.0　Written Change Control Policy; Includes Version Control

7.0　Archival Records

8.0　Security Practices—regarding unauthorized access and/or
　　　changes to source code

9.0　Documentation Practices

10.0　Documentation Provided to User (User's Guide)

11.0　Training Programs for Users

12.0　Availability of Source Code

13.0　Version Support Policies

14.0　Backup and Contingency Practices

15.0　Review of Software to be Purchased

　　15.01　Review of Source Code for Compliance with Standards
　　　　　　and Practices
　　15.02　Review of Archival History and Change Control
　　15.03　Review of Testing Records
　　15.04　Market History
　　15.05　Compatible with Functional Requirements and System
　　　　　　Specifications

audit trail with regard to document dating, use of a protocol supplement page is recommended. A single page that references the original protocol and states the reason for the change and the manner in which it will be executed is then reviewed and approved by the same authorities who approved the protocol. All protocol supplements are then attached to the original protocol in the file, presenting a complete and chronologically logical package.

Completion Reports

As almost any validation effort approaches completion, whether on schedule or behind, there is usually considerable interest in getting the system on-line and into productive use. That places completion of final reports and sign-offs on the critical path. A well-organized documentation system can help considerably in expediting things at this usually tense phase of the validation life cycle.

The Task Report is a collection of documents generated during execution of a Qualification Protocol (IQ, OQ, or PQ). An index that precisely identifies each document, including revision numbers, dates, titles, and so on, is essential. If the documents are not all physically together, location of each should also be identified.

A Task Report Summary (or Task Report Cover Page) is a useful vehicle, the purpose of which is to identify the exact protocol(s) executed, summarize the results and conclusions, and formally establish that the conclusions have been properly approved. A well-designed Cover, linked to an accurately indexed Task Report, can often satisfy the need for obtaining all approval signatures on a single page.

The Validation Completion Report is a comprehensive summary that explains how requirements of the Validation Project Plan have been satisfied. By referencing all relevant Task Report Summaries and the Validation Project Plan, the Completion Report can be kept brief, and also serve as a collection vehicle for all necessary signatures approving the total project.

Change Control Documents

Throughout any validation life cycle, many kinds of changes occur—to hardware, software, documents, and even assigned personnel. Since most validation documents are highly specific, it is important to have systems in place that treat changes formally, expeditiously, and accurately.

The validation life cycle starts with initial design and extends throughout the life of a system. In the early stages of a life cycle, change control practices can be inhibiting if overly formalized. In later stages, the importance of such formalities, such as approval by the quality control unit, often increases, in some cases even representing regulatory requirements. It is helpful to define

1. At what point in the life cycle formal change control is to begin; and

2. What change management measures are to be taken prior to that point.

Figure 4.2 illustrates a common approach for dealing with item 1.

Change management refers to practices employed for keeping information reasonably up-to-date in a manner not requiring formal approvals. For example, some firms with efficient electronic document management systems, use formal change control from the start of the life cycle. Many other firms, however, rely on "redlining" of drawings and wiring diagrams, and other such informal measures early in the project.

An important point to consider is that the validation project will benefit if even informal change management practices are described in policies or SOPs. Sooner or later, accurate information will be needed. The more "informal" changes that are allowed to accumulate in the early stages, the more difficult and time-consuming it may be to set the record straight later on, as qualification efforts begin. Hence, change management practices based on common sense ways of recording all changes not only helps economize on resources, but also minimizes tie-ups on the critical path later in the validation project.

Software change control is a well-established practice with most software suppliers that includes some features possibly applicable to other areas of change control. For example, it is common to define the following three categories of change:

1. *Cosmetic Changes*—those that do not affect operation of a computer-related system (e.g., spelling correction)

2. *Minor Changes*—those that affect only one section, or module, of a software program (e.g., change in a report layout), thus lending themselves to modular requalification

3. *Major Changes*—those that impact large portions of the system, thereby requiring full performance requalification

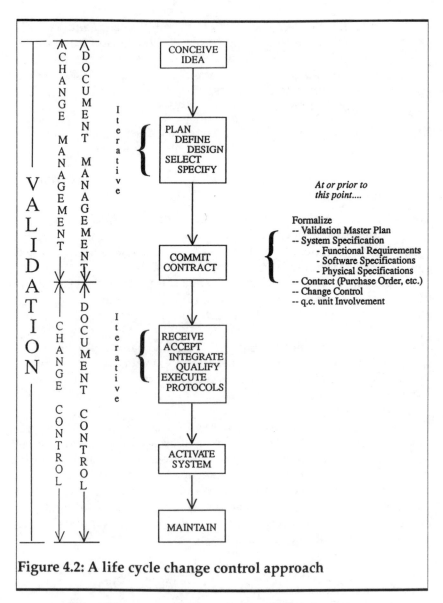

Figure 4.2: A life cycle change control approach

Analogous treatment of change control might be usefully applied to almost any system.

Document Change Control is usually simpler than software change control, but no less important. A key consideration is to ensure that everyone who uses the document for decision-making always has the correct version. A common mistake here is to assume that, so long as the latest documents are transmitted to all who need them, the documents will also be received, stored, and made retrievable in a reliable manner. The opposite is often true. To avoid this pitfall, it behooves the Validation Project Manager to establish a system early in the project that includes features such as those described on pages 54–55.

Periodic audits of all manuals, manual holder reassignments reflecting personnel changes, and careful attention to use of revision numbers and dates, can all contribute to an efficient and economic document management system.

WHAT'S MISSING?

No matter how thoroughly the documentation task is pursued, there is always the final nagging question, "Have I addressed everything that is required?" One might expect the answer to be difficult, especially if multiple geographical areas and various regulations are involved. Once again, the answer can be simplified by following a common sense approach. Appendices C, D, and E (pages 281–299) illustrate ways of correlating worldwide regulations using a checklist of basic validation concepts.

REFERENCES

1. Commission of the European Communities, "Computerized Systems," *Annex 11 to Good Manufacturing Practice for Medicinal Products in the European Community*, (January 1992).

2. Therapeutic Goods Administration, "Use of Computers," *Australian Code of GMP for Therapeutic Goods—Medicinal Products—Part 1* Section 9, (January 1993).

3. FDA, "Human and Veterinary Drugs, Current Good Manufacturing Practice in Manufacture, Processing, Packing or Holding," *Federal Register*, 43, No. 190, 45014–45089, (29 September 1978).

4. R. F. Tetzlaff, "GMP Documentation Requirements for Automated Systems: Part I" *Pharm. Technol.* 16 (3), 112–124; "Part II," *Pharm. Technol.* 16 (4), 60–72; and "Part III," *Pharm. Technol.* 16 (5), 70–83, (1992); also in *Pharm. Technol. Int.* 4 (5), (6), and (7), (1992).

5. K. G. Chapman, "A Procedural Approach to Quality Assurance," *Pharm. Tech. Conference 1982*, 45–60, (September 1982).

6. IEEE, "IEEE Std. 730-1989," *IEEE Standard for Software Quality Assurance Plans (ANSI)*, Institute of Electrical and Electronics Engineers, New York, (1989).

7. K. G. Chapman, "A History of Validation in the United States Part I," *Pharm. Technol.* 15 (10), 82–96, and "Part II, Validation of Computer-Related Systems," *Pharm. Technol.* 15 (11), 54–70, (1991).

8. PMA's Computer Systems Validation Committee, "Validation Concepts for Computer Systems Used in the Manufacture of Drug Products," *Pharm. Technol.* 10 (5), 24–34 (1986).

9. *International Standard ISO 9000-3*, "Quality Management and Quality Assurance Standards—Part 3: Guidelines for the Application of ISO 9001 to the Development, Supply and Maintenance of Software," International Organization for Standardization, Geneva, 1st ed., 1–15, (1991-06-01).

10. Parenteral Drug Association (PDA), "Validation of Computer-Related Systems," pre-publication monograph manuscript (October 1993).

11. A. J. Trill, "Computerized Systems and GMP—A UK Perspective: Part I Background, Standards and Methods," *Pharm. Technol. International* 5 (2), 12–26; "Part II Inspection Findings," *Pharm. Technol. International* 5 (3), 49–63; and "Part III Best Practices and Topical Issues," *Pharm. Technol. International* 5 (5), 17–30, (1993).

12. A. J. Trill, "A Medicines Inspector's Views on Validation Requirements for Computerized Systems in the European Drug Processing Industry," *Pharma. Technologie Journal* 11 (3), 86–89 (1990). Paper presented at the Concept-Symposium's "Validierung von Computersystemen in der Pharma-Industrie" 16–17 October 1990, Frankfurt am Main, Germany.

Appendix 4.1: Illustrative Table of Contents for a LIMS Validation Project Plan

---

1. System overview [*may include graphics to illustrate how the LIMS module fits into the total picture*]

2. LIM System Preliminary Definition

    2.1 Functional Requirements [*a preliminary definition of major perceived functions, based on earlier review with proposed Application Experts (end users)*]

    2.2 Physical Description [*e.g., preliminary description of probable layout of suitable PCs, file-servers, networks, and the like*]

    2.3 Software Requirements [*e.g., preliminary specification of the operating system, executive programs, canned configurables, and application code that are expected to be used*]

3. Validation Team Organization

    3.1 LIMS Validation Team

        3.1.1 Members, Chair, Secretary, QC Unit, Document Administrator, QA Auditor, et al

        3.1.2 Responsibilities

        3.1.3 Mission and Modus Operandi

    3.2 Related CIM Project Validation Teams

    3.3 Overall CIM Project Management Team

4. Timing and Scheduling

    4.1 Total CIM Project [*preliminary schedule with time landmarks*]

    4.2 LIMS Validation [*preliminary schedule with time landmarks that coincide appropriately with 4.1*]

5. Documentation Planning [*any or all of this section may be covered by existing policies/SOPs, which might be simply referenced*]

    5.1 Document Control System

    5.2 Review and Approval Process for

        5.2.1 Software QA Plans

        5.2.2 IQ Protocols, Reports, and Supplements

        5.2.3 OQ Protocols, Reports, and Supplements

        5.2.4 PQ Protocols, Reports, and Supplements

        5.2.5 Documentation Change Controls

        5.2.6 Physical System Change Controls

Continued on next page

6. Software QA Planning *[any or all of this section may be covered by existing policies/SOPs, which may be simply referenced]*

    6.1 Assurance of Structural Integrity

        6.1.1 By Vendor SQA Audits

        6.1.2 By In-House SQA Audits

        6.1.3 By researching specific version market histories

    6.2 Functional Testing—Planned Approaches

        6.2.1 Modular basis (LIMS)

        6.2.2 LIMS—integrated

        6.2.3 CIM—integrated

    6.3 Consultants and System Integrators

        6.3.1 Potential Roles

        6.3.2 Liaison Arrangements with LIMS Team(s)

        6.3.3 Documentation of Credentials

7. Security *[any or all of this section may be covered by existing policies/SOPs, which may be simply referenced]*

    7.1 Password Control

    7.2 Physical Access Control

    7.3 Virus Prevention

    7.4 Data Backup, Retention, Retrieval

    7.5 Protection of Data Transmission and Reception

8. System Change Control and Revalidation *[any or all of this section may be covered by existing policies/SOPs, which may be simply referenced]*

    8.1 Hardware Changes

    8.2 Software Changes

    8.3 Document Changes

9. Recovery and Contingency Plans

    9.1 Periodic Test Protocols and Schedules

5

Validation Concepts
and Key Terminology

Kenneth G. Chapman
Director, Systems and Planning
Corporate Quality Assurance Audit
Pfizer Inc.
Groton, CT, USA

The rate at which we learn is a function of the size and depth of our vocabulary. The rate at which validation concepts become established is also governed largely by the rate at which associated terminology evolves and is accepted.

All of the above processes are dynamic. Historically, several difficult validation issues have been resolved as the direct result of new validation terminology or the acceptance of new definitions after deliberation. Such landmark progress occurred only after the U.S. industry and the FDA attained agreement on terms like *worst case* and *edge-of-failure* in 1984–86, *canned configurables* and *structural integrity* in 1987, and *electronic signatures* in 1993.

This chapter provides insight to some historic, recent, current, and possibly future, terminology changes and offers what this author deems to be the "best" contemporary definitions for several key terms. Definitions discussed below are provided in Tables 5.1–5.5 and in Appendix 2.

Even the authors of different chapters in this book may use slightly different terms or interpretations, partially due to native language variations, but mostly because of today's still dynamic evolution of validation terminology.

SOME KEY TERMS

Validation

Validation has probably been redefined by half the authors who have written about the subject in the last two decades. Prior to 1983, the FDA's definition was clear and simple: *Establishing documented evidence that a system does what it purports to do.* Most authors, including this one in a 1983 article, "A Suggested Validation Lexicon" (1), adopted the FDA's definition, applying it to the validation of manufacturing and water treatment processes and computer systems through 1986 (2–5).

In 1987, the FDA offered an expanded definition for process validation [Table 5.1] that quickly became popular and continues in wide current use: *Process validation is establishing documented evidence that provides a high degree of assurance that a specific process will consistently produce a product meeting its predetermined specifications and quality attributes.* Most other categories of validation in the United States have definitions patterned after this definition.

Table 5.1: Process Validation	
FDA before 1983	**FDA after 1987**
Establishing documented evidence that a system does what it purports to do	*Establishing documented evidence that provides a high degree of assurance that a specific process will consistently produce a product meeting its predetermined specifications and quality attributes*

Several important concepts are embedded in the FDA's 1987 definition. "Documented evidence," already part of the earlier definition, had been misinterpreted by some to mean "proof." To reemphasize the FDA's awareness that absolute proof is unachievable, the words *a high degree of assurance* were included. Other key embedded concepts include the following:

- The process must be specific (i.e., clearly defined).

- The process must be consistent and reproducible.

- Process functions must be predefined in ways that identify specifications and quality attributes of the product being manufactured.

In recent years, the authors of the 1986 Pharmaceutical Manufacturers' Association (PMA) concept paper for computer system validation (6) realized that two definitions used in its validation life cycle presentation conflicted somewhat with each other and required clarification: *validation plan* and *validation protocol*. In the plan, *validation* embraces all phases of the system or process being addressed; in the protocol, it refers only to the specific experimental step following Operational Qualification (OQ). Contemporary U.S. industry thinking has led to replacing the latter step with the term *Performance Qualification (PQ)*. Thus, the familiar Validation Protocol should ultimately disappear. The *Validation Project Plan*, discussed in chapter 4, now embraces the entire project. The Validation Timeline in Figure 5.1 illustrates use of this latest terminology.

Another example concerning various meanings of validation is the IEEE definition: *The process of evaluating software at the end of the software development process to ensure compliance with software requirements*. (7) Since IEEE specifically addresses only the software aspects of computer-related system validation, the definition represents an appropriate use of the term validation. It probably appears inconsistent, however, with the definition used for the subject of this book, both of which address the total system.

A fundamental purpose of all validation in the healthcare industry is to protect fitness-for-use of its end products [Table 5.2]. Unfortunately, some consulting firms define validation today in a manner that is self-serving, using the term for everything from plant architecture to landscaping. The reader is advised to be wary of such "consultants" and remember, "don't let them validate the pencil sharpeners!"

Table 5.2: Fitness-for-Use of Finished Products

• Safety	• Stability
• Efficacy	• Identity
• Purity	• [Elegance]
• Strength	

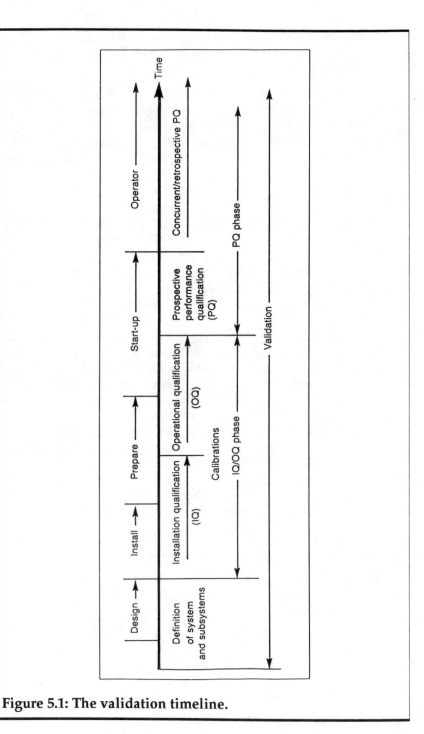

Figure 5.1: The validation timeline.

Computer, Computerized, and Computer-Related Systei.

Most readers have probably experienced some confusion bet~
terms like *software validation, computer validation, computer system val~.
tion,* and *computerized system validation.* Actually, all four are meaning
ful terms, yet none represents the most common subject of today's
validation project planning, which is *computer-related system validation.*

Figure 5.2 illustrates all five terms. Software represents part of a
computer and the IEEE definition of validation satisfies that application. The computer system, which includes some peripheral hardware
as well as software, can be validated by itself, although in today's vernacular, it would more likely be "qualified." The computerized system
includes those processes and subsystems (hardware and/or software)
that are directly controlled by the computer; again, the computerized
system can be "qualified" and/or "validated."

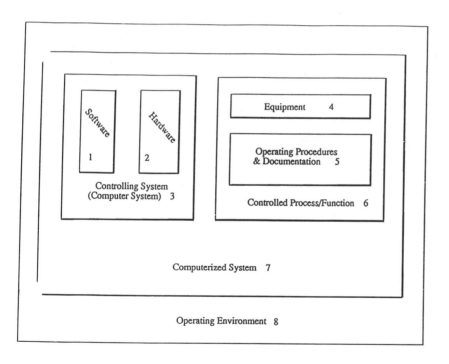

COMPUTER-RELATED SYSTEM   9

Figure 5.2: Five key phrases.

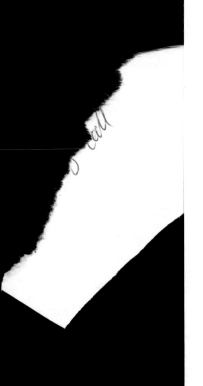

Most computerized systems in today's world of CIM, LIMS, and MRP (see Appendix 1) are affected by the surrounding *Operating Environment*, which often includes other computerized systems. For the total system to be in a state of control, all related systems (and subsystems) must also be in a state of control, which usually means *Qualified* or *Validated*. Thus, the total system, which consists of the computerized system plus its operating environment, is referred to as a *Computer-Related System*, the primary subject of most validation project planning today.

Figure 5.3 depicts an Operating Environment surrounding a typical LIM (Laboratory Information Management) System to further illustrate the *Computer-Related System* concept. Let us assume that the LIMS has been "fully qualified," which means documented evidence has been gathered that indicates everything is satisfactory. Note that some relational database information and some direct digital data from an HPLC (High Pressure Liquid Chromatography) instrument are fed into the LIMS. If these two external systems are already qualified and in a state of validated control, the only thing new that is needed in the Validation Project Plan will be the interfaces with LIMS; conversely, if either of the subsystems has not already received validation attention, such effort becomes part of the Validation Project Plan.

Also note the two pH meters. In one case, an operator reads the meter and enters the original data directly into the LIMS computer database using a terminal. In the second case, an operator records the data on a pad, after which another person, perhaps a data entry clerk, transcribes the data using a terminal. Here, for the total system to become validated, it will be necessary to establish that the pH meters are not only properly maintained, buffered, and calibrated, but also that approved SOPs exist for operating the pH meter and for transcribing, entering, and verifying data, that the operators' training is adequate and documented, and so on. In other words, validation planning should address everything that must be done to bring the *Computer-Related System* into a state of control.

Functional Requirements Versus Physical Description

Nowhere has the need for consistent terminology become more apparent than in the area of defining the purpose of the system that is to be validated. It is more than coincidence that most new project failures involving computer-related systems stem directly from failure to adequately predict the system's *Functional Requirements*.

The issue in this case results not from a lack of defined terms (if anything, there are too many), but rather from a failure to appreciate

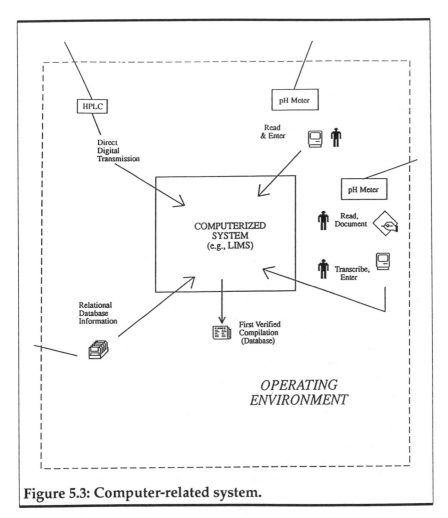

Figure 5.3: Computer-related system.

the need for a multidisciplinary team that communicates effectively. While the computer scientist certainly represents a key discipline, an even more important one for defining functional requirements is the end user, who might more appropriately be referred to as an "application expert."

Some firms have developed a practice of grouping functional requirements and physical requirements together under the term *functional specifications*. For projects involving only software, such terminology would be consistent with IEEE definitions and nonproblematical; however, for the type of multidisciplinary teams demanded by computer-related system validation, such vernacular can lead to omissions and confusion.

It is recommended that the definition of *Functional Requirements* be given the highest priority at the project start, and that the definition not be compromised by including any physical requirements or specification data (such as operating systems, hardware to be used, or the number of pixels on the screen). In the preceding chapter, Figure 4.1 illustrated the typical development sequence of *functional requirements, system definition*, and *system specifications*. Such development is iterative and highly dependent on the quality of the *Functional Requirements* document.

Software Quality Issues

In the early 1980s computer scientists and programmers represented the only disciplines that understood how to assure software quality; the language they used was foreign to most other disciplines. As rapid evolution of new technology inexorably led to GMP-related computer applications in the United States, the "QC unit" responsible for assurance of quality found itself needing to become computer literate enough to also understand the subject. By the mid-1980s, the important question was no longer how to develop reliable software, but rather how to purchase reliable software. This called for a team from the user-firm to work with the software supplier—a team that could, at least collectively, understand the language and the technology of software quality assurance.

It soon became apparent that it was not enough for a programming group to simply say it "followed the IEEE standards"; auditors found that programmers often worked from memory and were unable to even find the standards. Auditors from pharmaceutical firms felt that written software development procedures were needed [Table 4.3].

The 1987 publication of Compliance Policy Guide 7132a.15 (8) brought several issues into focus. It called for source code inspection, raising the question, "To what extent should quality be tested and inspected into, rather than built into, software?" As the result of deliberation aimed at answering this question, the industry and the FDA discovered the importance of a category of software previously unrecognized or defined.

Two general categories of software programs had been defined by IEEE (9), by FDA (10), and by PMA (11):

1. System software, which includes the operating system

2. Application software [Table 5.3]

Table 5.3: Software Types

Application Software: Software specifically produced for the functional use of a computer system

Operating System: Software that controls the execution of programs

---

FDA and PMA principals agreed that source code possession and inspections were appropriate for application software. It was also unofficially agreed that operating system software, which is exercised every time the application program is run, could be purchased and used on the basis of demonstrated market performance.

A closer scrutiny then revealed that a new, undefined software category had emerged to dominate the marketplace; this category, now referred to as the *Canned Configurable* (12, 13), is discussed in chapter 4, portrayed in Figure 5.4, and defined in Appendix 2.

The source code deliberation also caused the industry to develop a better understanding of *structural and functional* software testing requirements. It became apparent that, when the needs for structural testing are shown to have been satisfied, remaining validation can be based on functional testing alone (14).

The U.S. military uses the acronym COTS, for "Commercial Off-the-Shelf" software, a term nearly identical to *Canned Configurable*. Purchase of COTS software is based on rigorous Department of Defense (DoD) standards, which adequately address both the structural and functional testing aspects of software quality assurance.

Boundary Values, Worst Case, and Edge-of-Failure

In software parlance, "boundary values" relates to "stress testing" [Table 5.4] and can be related to a phrase used with process validation, known as *worst case*. This phrase has proven to be one of the most problematic in the history of validation in the United States. Defining "worst case" required 2 years of deliberation between the FDA and the U.S. pharmaceutical industry, the results of which can be grasped in about 2 minutes by studying Figure 5.5.

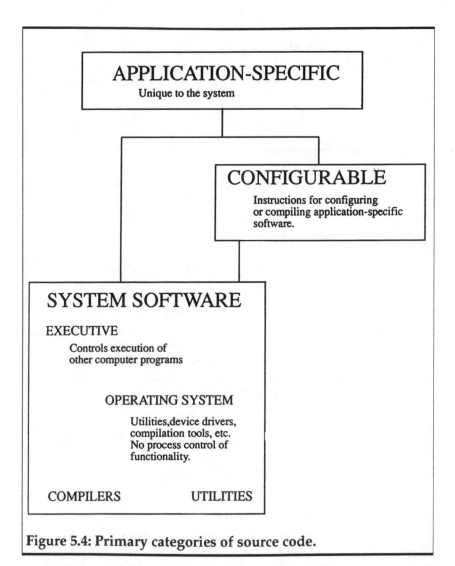

Figure 5.4: Primary categories of source code.

Table 5.4: Validation Parameters

Boundary Value: A data value that corresponds to a minimum or maximum input, internal, or output value specified for a system or component (15)

Stress Testing: Testing conducted to evaluate a system or component at or beyond the limits of its specified requirements (16)

Edge-of-Failure: A control parameter value that, if exceeded, means adverse effect on state of control and/or fitness for use of the product (17)

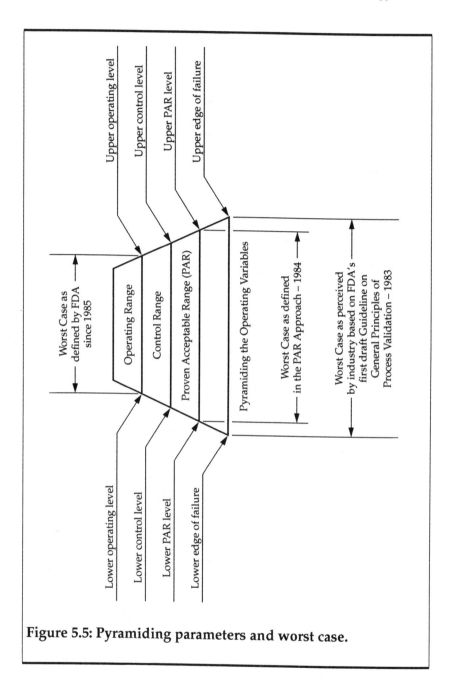

Figure 5.5: Pyramiding parameters and worst case.

In 1983 the FDA stated that process validation should " . . . include worst case challenges of the process." (18) At the time, the FDA's unde-fined intentions were taken to mean that edge-of-failure conditions had to be identified and included in large-scale runs in order to validate a process. In 1984 this author suggested another definition for "worst case" in "The PAR (Proven Acceptable Range) Approach to Process Validation" (19), acceptance of which would make it unnecessary to establish, or even encounter, edge-of-failure values. Finally, the FDA decided in 1985 that process validation efforts need only establish acceptability of the actual operating range as stated in a firm's manufacturing instructions; a position that was later formalized in FDA's final version of its 1987 guideline (20) (see Table 5.3).

Definitions of "worst case" and "boundary conditions" are important because the terms represent key values to be established in most validation efforts. The five basic steps of validating a process include

1. Identify the "Critical Process Parameters."

2. Identify the approximate "Critical Process Parameter Ranges" to be established (target boundary conditions).

3. Define the potential adverse consequences of exceeding the range (beyond each upper and lower boundary condition).

4. Gather data, prospectively or retrospectively, to support the boundary conditions.

5. Establish process reproducibility ("robustness").

Retrospective, Prospective, and Concurrent Validation

The words *retrospective* and *retroactive* are almost, but not quite, identical. Some authors have trouble recognizing the difference; however, when these terms relate to validation, an important distinction exists. This author regards *retroactive* process validation as occurring after product made by the process has been released for human or animal use. *Retrospective* process validation, however, should be considered unrelated to the commercial or clinical status of the product. [Table 5.5]

To appreciate the significance of these validation terms, it is worth recognizing there are two general categories of data basic to process validation:

1. Data to establish robustness and reproducibility of the full-scale process

2. Data to provide evidence that boundary conditions of all critical process parameter ranges are acceptable

The first category requires multiple, successful, production-size batches. The second category might involve prospective efforts, such as

---

Table 5.5: Validation Types

Prospective Validation: Establishing documented evidence that a system does what it purports to do based on a validation plan

Concurrent Process Validation: Establishing documented evidence that a process does what it purports to do based on information generated during actual implementation of the process

Retrospective Validation: Establishing documented evidence that a system does what it purports to do based on review and analysis of historic information

Retroactive Validation: Establishing documented evidence that a system does what it purports to do after the system is used for commercial purposes

---

physicochemical profiles generated in a physical pharmacy laboratory, or retrospective efforts that incorporate existing data from routine batch records, investigation reports, R&D documents, and even laboratory and pilot plant experiments. Such retrospective data are often significant and abundantly available; not only for a process that has been in production for years, but also for a process whose product may still be in Phase II clinical trials. Retrospective process validation is, therefore, useful when establishing changes to a well-established process, and when conducting process validation for a new product.

Sterilization validation and aseptic process validation must be conducted prospectively, since both are premised on the point that the quality attribute known as sterility cannot be determined by end-product testing alone. In the case of nonaseptic process validation, a different situation exists. Many quality attributes, unlike sterility, do lend themselves to accurate determination by end-product testing, provided validated sampling plans and analytical test methods are used. Thus, many validation situations lend themselves to the retrospective approach.

Concurrent process validation has also been historically confusing, and even controversial. Although less frequently used, concurrent validation is essential for orphan drugs and certain clinical supply situations where limited material is available. Water treatment processes can also be used to illustrate concurrent validation and its relationship to prospective approaches (21, 22). As depicted in Figure 5.1, once prospective evidence is gathered to show that the system performs properly, it is reasonable to start using the water for clinical or commercial purposes. Frequency of testing and monitoring is usually higher during the early concurrent phase, since system performance and indigenous bioburden might be affected by seasonal and other long-term factors. As experience grows, and the long-term effects are understood, testing needs become better defined until the system can be finally declared validated.

Process validation is important to computer-related system validation, because no system involving process control can be validated unless the process being controlled is itself validated.

Electronic Signatures

From August 1990 through late 1993, many deliberations occurred in the United States concerning use of *electronic signatures* and *electronic identifications*. Resolution of most issues once again revolved around semantics and definitions of terminology (23, 24). Such resolution appears near at hand as this book is being completed, with terminology and definitions still being finalized.

The future of nearly all paperless operations, including electronic batch records, as well as CIM, LIMS, and MRP applications, depends on use of electronic signatures. Hence, reaching agreement on concepts and terminology represents a matter of worldwide urgency.

Expert Systems

At a meeting in July 1992, PMA's Computer System Validation Committee addressed the question, "Can expert systems be validated?" The group's initial responses were evenly divided between affirmative and negative. As it turned out, both answers were correct. The issue turned out to be another useful example of the important role terminology can play in developing conceptual understanding.

Experience had already underscored the importance of semantics, so the committee proceeded by first defining *Expert System*. Deliberations revealed that expert systems fall into two basic categories:

1. Those in which the rules and related databases can change without human intervention, as experience grows

2. Those in which such changes can be made only with human intervention

Further discussion led to the conclusions that category 2 above can be qualified (i.e., "validated"); but, category 1 probably cannot, since unpredictability of "correct" test results renders functional testing impossible.

GLP (Good Laboratory Practices)

Since 1976, the FDA has used the term *GLP* to mean good laboratory practices that relate to nonclinical laboratory studies (i.e., those that involve product safety and toxicity experiments with various species of animals). Most other regulatory agencies worldwide have adopted similar meanings for the GLP acronym. Even today, newcomers to this somewhat restrictive use of GLP are confused when they discover it is not intended to cover other laboratories, such as those involved in GMP applications.

In 1990, the U.S. EPA (Environmental Protection Agency) published a draft guideline on Good Automated Lab Practices (25), using the acronym *GALP* to embrace all laboratories. In hindsight, the FDA might have done better to adopt a more descriptive acronym, such as GNCPs, for "Good Nonclinical Practices." The case provides another useful example of the importance of selecting appropriate terms and acronyms.

GCP (Good Clinical Practices)

The term *protocol* might serve as a final example that illustrates the importance of semantics. In validation parlance *protocol* represents a set of experimental directions, whereas a medical doctor who conducts clinical studies might consider a *protocol* something more analogous to the Validation Project Plan.

SUMMARY

Historically, progress in establishing universal, conceptual understanding of various forms of validation has been accelerated by agreement on key terminology definitions, and inhibited when guidelines or regulations lacking clear definitions are issued. Fortunately, most regulatory and standard-setting authorities today, as well as several technical and professional industrial associations, have recognized this need and are contributing toward worldwide harmonization of validation terms and concepts.

REFERENCES

1. K. G. Chapman, "A Suggested Validation Lexicon," *Pharm. Technol.* 7 (8), 51–57 (1983).

2. K. G. Chapman, "The PAR Approach to Process Validation," *Pharm. Technol.* 8 (12), 22–36 (1984).

3. PMA's Validation Advisory Committee, "Process Validation Concepts for Drug Products," *Pharm. Technol.* 9 (9), 78–82 (1985).

4. PMA's DIW Committee, "Validation and Control Concepts for Water Treatment Systems," *Pharm. Technol.* 9 (10), 50–56 (1985).

5. PMA's Computer Systems Validation Committee, "Validation Concepts for Computer Systems Used in the Manufacture of Drug Products," *Pharm. Technol.* 10 (5), 24–34 (1986).

6. Ibid.

7. IEEE, *IEEE Std. 610.2-1990*, "Glossary of Software Engineering Terminology (ANSI)," Institute of Electrical and Electronics Engineers, New York (1990).

8. FDA, Compliance Policy Guide on Computerized Drug Processing CPG 7132a.15, *Source Code for Process Control Application Programs*, April 1987.

9. IEEE Std. 610.2-1990.

10. FDA, "Guide to Inspection of Computerized Systems Used in the Manufacture of Drug Products," (the *BLUEBOOK*), Feb., 1983.

11. PMA, "Validation Concepts for Computer Systems Used in the Manufacture of Drug Products."

12. K. G. Chapman, et al., "Source Code Availability and Vendor-User Relationships," *Pharmaceutical Technology*, 11, (12), 24–35, December, 1987.

13. K. G. Chapman, "A History of Validation in the United States, Part I," *Pharm. Technol.* 15 (10), 82–96, and "Part II, Validation of Computer-Related Systems," *Pharm. Technol.* 15 (11), 54–70, (1991)

14. Ibid.

15. IEEE Std. 610.2-1990.

16. Ibid.

17. Chapman, "A Suggested Validation Lexicon."

18. *Guideline on General Principles of Process Validation—First Draft.* National Center for Drugs and Biologics and National Center for Devices and Radiological Health, Rockville, MD (March 1983).

19. Chapman, "The PAR Approach to Process Validation."

20. *Guideline on General Principles of Process Validation.* National Center for Drugs and Biologics and National Center or Devices and Radiological Health, Rockville, MD (May 15, 1987).

21. PMA, "Validation and Control Concepts for Water Treatment Systems."

22. Chapman, "A History of Validation in the United States, Part I" and "Part II, Validation of Computer-Related Systems."

23. P. J. Motise, "FDA Considerations on Electronic Identification and Signatures," *Pharm. Technol.* 16 (11), 29–35, 82 (1992).

24. K. G. Chapman & P. F. Winter, "Electronic Identification and Signatures: A Response," *Pharm. Technol.* 16 (11), 36–46, (1992).

25. Environmental Protection Agency (U.S. EPA) and Weinberg Associates, Inc. *Good Automated Lab Practices Implementation Manual,* (DRAFT) August, 1990.

26. A. J. Trill, "A Medicines Inspector's Views on Validation Requirements for Computerized Systems in the European Drug Processing Industry," *Pharma. Technologie Journal* 11 (3), 86–89 (1990). Paper presented at the Concept-Symposium's "Validierung von Computersystemen in der Pharma-Industrie" 16–17 October 1990, Frankfurt am Main, Germany.

6

Existing Computer Systems: A Practical Approach to Retrospective Evaluation

Dr. Heinrich Hambloch
European Consultant, Systems Validation
GITP: Good Information Technology Practices
Hofheim, Germany

Many of the computer systems used in the GXP area (X stands traditionally for C, L, and M) of pharmaceutical companies probably do not comply with the modern requirements for documentation and testing. This is not surprising because at the time many of the computer systems in use today were developed, the principles of quality assurance for software were not widely known.

On the other hand, conscientious programmers have always tested their modules and systems; unfortunately this has not been documented because there was no pressure to do it. So one cannot globally say that old computer systems are bad and that their use leads directly to disaster.

Technical progress alone cannot be a reason to throw away all the old computer systems and to replace them by modern ones, no more than a time-tested tablet machine is phased out when a new model is placed on the market. But, in the meantime, the authorities expect every computer system used in the GXP areas of pharmaceutical companies to be validated. There is no statement that old systems are excluded.

According to an FDA inspector:

There should be no question in anyone's mind, that FDA expects computer systems to be validated. (1)

And from a British inspector:

Action is required to bring these systems into agreement with the requirements of GMP. These will be concerned with the retrospective evaluation, modification and documentation of the systems to remedy the problems of noncompliance. (2)

The Red Apple Document has been worked out by representatives from the authorities, the pharmaceutical industry, and universities. On page 18 it states:

. . . there is general agreement that there needs to be a formal process for ensuring that these older systems are operating correctly. (3)

Apart from considerations in part 3 of Tony Trill's paper (4), there is very little in the literature concerning the validation or requalification of existing systems.

Therefore, the goal of this chapter is to develop a strategy for the retrospective evaluation of computer systems and to demonstrate the subsequent documenting and testing by means of a practical example. It is assumed that this system, a LIMS, has already been in use for a long time, is stable and reliable, and therefore will be used for another couple of years.

The author has applied this strategy several times in his practice in the pharmaceutical industry and later as a validation consultant. The method for retrospective evaluation described here is a practical and pragmatic approach to bring old computer systems into an acceptable status.

The term *retrospective evaluation* has been taken over from the Red Apple Document. It is used here instead of the term *retrospective validation* just to differentiate the technique described here from the validation techniques applied to the development of new computer systems. The term *validation* should be reserved for systems developed according to the System Development Life Cycle (SDLC).

A STRATEGY FOR RETROSPECTIVE EVALUATION

The retrospective evaluation of a computer system can be divided into the following phases:

- Preparation of an experience report

- Collection of all available documentation and assessment of its quality

- Determination of GXP-relevant functions

- Cost estimate for evaluation and decision on continuing use of the system

- Updating the document(s) used for testing

- Testing the system

- Risk assessment

- Formal release

Some of these activities and documents could be summarized under the title *validation plan*. However, this process uses the term *retrospective evaluation* instead of *retrospective validation* so the term *evaluation plan* is more appropriate. In the following section the activities performed during the several phases of retrospective evaluation will be described in detail.

THE PHASES OF RETROSPECTIVE EVALUATION

Preparation of an Experience Report

An experience report can be very helpful in making the decision whether or not to continue further use and development of the computer system. Such a report can show the decision makers the following:

- When and by whom and with which tools the system has been developed

- How far quality assurance concepts have been applied

- How widespread is the use of the software in industry

- Where the software is used within the company

- Who are the users of the software

- How often the main functions are used

- Where problems have occurred in the past

The purpose of the experience report is to show the degree of maturity and stability of the computer system, which are also quality criteria of the system.

Collection of Documentation and Assessment of Its Quality

After the preparation of the experience report, all the available documentation of the system should be collected. The documentation usually consists of the following:

The System Specification

The specification describes the system from the user's point of view (e.g., what should the system do). All inputs, outputs, processing steps, calculations, and interfaces to other systems are characterized in the system specification document.

The System Design Manual

The manual describes the system from the programmer's point of view (e.g., how should the system do it). Here the data models, their translation into file and database structures, screen and report layouts, and interfaces are listed in detail.

The Source Code

The source code contains the computer instructions in the form of a programming language or in the form of parameter settings of 4 GL tools, respectively.

The Installation Manual

The manual describes the installation on a target computer and the necessary software and hardware resources (e.g., the required operating system, compiler, database system, printers, etc.).

The User Manual

The user manual explains the use of all functions of the computer system as well as its limits in the user's language.

The nomenclature of the above documents and the distribution of their contents over the documents varies from system to system and from company to company. Here it is only important that the described contents are covered by the respective documents.

Depending on the complexity of the system, other documents may be available. Regarding process control systems, in addition to the above mentioned documents, there are usually construction plans, specifications of special hardware parts like valves and thermometers, calibration instructions, wiring diagrams, and so on.

After collecting the available documents, their quality must be assessed. It must be investigated, if the documents actually reflect the current status of the system. This phase requires great experience in the field of quality assurance and should only be carried out by properly trained data-processing professionals.

Today a number of companies have SOPs for the structure and the content of the documentation required for the development of new computer systems. These SOPs are also useful for the retrospective evaluation, because they can serve as checklists and can therefore provide a structured approach to the examination of the documentation of these old systems.

After assessing the quality of the documentation, the document(s) best suited for the derivation of the tests should be chosen. Usually these are the following documents:

- The system specification

- The system design manual

- The user manual

In practice, however, often not all of these documents are available, or the documents are not up-to-date. In this case, the document that can be updated in the simplest way should be chosen as the basic document for the derivation of the tests. In many cases this is the user manual. If changes in the system are intended for the future, then the system manual must be brought up-to-date as well.

When the most suitable document has been chosen, the costs for bringing it into an acceptable condition should be estimated. Such a cost estimate will help a company make the decision whether or not to continue using the system in the future.

Determination of GXP-Relevant Functions

In order to limit the effort for the retrospective evaluation to the really necessary proportion that is required to guarantee drug safety, only the functions that affect the GXPs must be evaluated. These functions are determined via the GXP analysis. By this analysis it is determined, if a function

- Has influence on the pharmaceutical technical quality.

- Affects the medical safety of the drug.

- Has influence on the data that become part of the registration documents.

- Is critical because of another important reason.

The following example explains this method by means of a Laboratory Information and Management System (LIMS) in a production environment. Some of the LIMS functions with GXP relevance are as follows:

- The correct transmission of data from analytical instruments

- The correct transmission of the release status to the stock system

- The correct transmission of the results on the Certificate of Analysis

- The transmission only of validated methods to the instruments

- The correct check of analytical results against the predefined range limits

If a system function is to be excluded from retrospective evaluation, this exclusion must be justified in writing. Taking a LIMS as an example, the following functions certainly do not have to be evaluated:

- Cross-charging the client for analytical work

- The distribution of the workload on different laboratories

- The monitoring of the time a sample is in the laboratory

- The statistics about the number of Karl-Fischer analyses in 1987

These functions are of operational nature only and do not affect the quality of analytical results.

The GXP analysis requires a great level of experience and should be carried out by the GXP responsible person. The most suitable documents to use for identifying the GXP-relevant functions are the system specification and the user manual. This is because they are written in the user's language, in contrast to the system design manual that contains the programming details.

Costs Estimates and Decision on Continued Use of the System

On the basis of the

- Experience report,

- Effort to bring the documentation up-to-date, and

- GXP analysis,

an estimate can be made of the cost for doing the retrospective evaluation. Then a business decision can be made about whether it is worthwhile to conduct the whole evaluation process or whether it is more cost-effective on a long-term basis to introduce a new computer system.

For the rest of this evaluation procedure, it is assumed that the computer system in question remains in use and will not be changed in the future.

Review of the Document Used for Testing

In the revision phase of retrospective evaluation, the document selected for the derivation of the tests must be brought up-to-date. The choice of the user manual for this purpose has three advantages:

- It has to be in place and up-to-date anyway.

- It clearly describes all functions of the computer system.

- It is written in the user's language and therefore facilitates the GXP analysis.

The review of the user manual takes place while all the functions of the computer system are executed at a terminal. If it is intended to modify the system in the future, the system design manual should also be updated to an acceptable status.

Testing the System

Testing the system is in many cases the most labor-intensive phase in retrospective evaluation and requires a careful planning of all activities, which are described in a document called the Test Plan. Before such a Test Plan can be developed, it should be made clear which of the many quality attributes of the system are to be tested.

Table 6.1 lists the most important quality attributes of a computer system. All these attributes can be tested. But what is of most interest here is testing the functionality of the computer system against a writ-

Table 6.1: Quality Attributes of a Computer System		
Safety	**Maintainability**	**Usability**
reliable	restorable	stable
access-safe	modifiable	self-explanatory
recoverable		user-friendly
		resource-friendly
		meets specifications

ten description. This, and only this, is required by the following commonly accepted definition of validation, derived from a PMA paper:

> Validation is the documented evidence that a computer system does what it purports to do and continues to do so. (5)

This leads directly to a definition of testing, used in a major firm:

> Testing is the always repeatable proof of the correct functioning of a computer system according to predetermined requirements. Testing does not mean to execute a computer system in order to find errors.

The latter is impossible per se because the errors that are searched for are unfortunately not known in advance. Therefore, by all logic, it is impossible to search for things that are unknown.

In order to find all errors by testing the computer system, all the possible combinations of paths would have to be executed with all possible combinations of data—an absolutely impractical undertaking. A few years ago, this demand wandered like a ghost through the literature relevant to the subject. An example of the impracticability of this unstructured procedure is given in *The Art of Software Testing*. (6)

On the grounds of these disadvantages, the first part of the testing definition is followed, namely the test against a written description. In many cases of retrospective evaluation, the user manual can be used as the written description.

In contrast to the pragmatic approach for the retrospective evaluation described here, it should be clear that the design and development of a new computer system should consider all of the quality attributes described in Table 6.1.

After these more theoretical comments, the testing will be described in detail. As is usual in the pharmaceutical community, this should be done in the form of an SOP. An SOP, which describes the construction, execution, and documentation of test plans is shown in Figure 6.1.

Risk Assessment

Risk assessment describes which GXP functions influenced by the computer system are still critical, even after the testing. A reasonable safety of these functions should be accomplished by other arrangements such as establishing organizational precautions.

Formal Release

The release document formally releases the computer system as having satisfactorily completed retrospective evaluation. From now on all future system changes must be carried out only in accordance with a change control procedure and with an updated system design manual at hand.

A PRACTICAL EXAMPLE

Having defined all the necessary steps for retrospective evaluation, a practical example is now carried out according to the SOP for the Retrospective Testing of Computer Systems (Figure 6.1). A LIMS has been chosen as the computer system example and it is assumed that it collects and evaluates data from routine analyses performed in a pharmaceutical production environment (i.e., the system affects the GMPs).

The document from which the tests are derived is the User Manual and it is assumed that the User Manual has already been updated. Figure 6.2 shows the part of the User Manual that is relevant for the derivation of the tests to provide the manual data input function in this example.

The GXP analysis has shown that the manual input of analytical results can affect the GMPs, because errors in the manual data input can lead to erroneous batch releases. This can occur if input data outside the range limit are not recognized by the system.

Furthermore it is assumed that the testing of this function has not been covered yet by other preceding tests. Thus the function *Manual Data Input* has to be marked in the user manual with blue color and numbered according to the SOP TEST/001.

The test cases derived from this part of the User Manual are shown in Figure 6.3. Figure 6.4 contains the test goals for test case 4. Figure 6.5

shows the test instructions for test goal 2. The test plan, which consists of Figures 6.3–6.5 is now complete with respect to test case 4, test goal 2. It should be examined and signed by a second competent person.

Now the tests can be carried out and documented according to the Test Plan. In this example the documentation consists of a screen copy that can be stored as an electronic file or printed out on paper. The completed test documentation for test case 4, test goal 2 is shown in Figure 6.6. In the same way the other test goals and test instructions must be developed, carried out, and documented.

CONCLUSION

In this chapter a structured approach to the retrospective evaluation of existing computer systems has been demonstrated using a test SOP in conjunction with a practical example. It is a pragmatic approach based on personal experience, and known to work.

Regarding the effort for such an approach, experience has shown that database systems of this kind (LIMS, PPS, EBRS, etc.) require several hundred test cases with possibly several thousand test instructions. The development and execution of these tests can add up to 0.5–3 years of work depending on the size of the system.

Therefore, it should be carefully checked whether the cost of the retrospective evaluation is in fact worthwhile or whether it is more cost-effective to introduce a new computer system for the regulated function.

Figure 6.1: SOP for the Retrospective Testing of Computer Systems

< Name of the Company>
Standard Operating Procedure TEST/001

Retrospective Testing of Computer Systems
Valid from: 01.01.93   Version 2.2   Page 1 of 6

Prepared by:

_____ / _____ <NAME, DEPT.>
Signature   Date
(signs for correctness and completeness)

Approved by:

1._____ / _____ <NAME, DEPT.>
Signature   Date
(signs for control of correctness and completeness)

2. _____ / _____ <NAME, DEPT.>
Signature   Date
(signs for conformity with GXP guidelines)

Released by:

1. _____ / _____ <NAME, DEPT>
Signature   Date
(signs for release of SOP)

Continued on next page

Figure 6.1 continued

< Name of the Company>
Standard Operating Procedure TEST/001

Retrospective Testing of Computer Systems

Valid from: 01.01.93   Version 2.2   Page 2 of 6

Table of contents

1   General

    1.1   Purpose

    1.2   Principle

    1.3   Validity

2   Procedure

    2.1   GXP analysis

    2.2   Test plan development

    2.3   Test execution and documentation

3   Distribution

4   Appendices

continued on next page

Figure 6.1 continued

< Name of the Company>
Standard Operating Procedure TEST/001

Retrospective Testing of Computer Systems
Valid from: 01.01.93   Version 2.2   Page 3 of 6

---

1 General

1.1 Purpose

The SOP *Retrospective Testing of Computer Systems* describes the development of a test plan, its execution and documentation, for the testing of existing computer systems.

1.2 Principles

Authority representatives require the evidence that old computer systems function according to the specifications (i.e., there is a demand for the retrospective evaluation of already existing computer systems).

1.3 Validity

This SOP is valid for all computer systems that potentially affect the GXPs (X stands traditionally for C, L, and M).

2 Procedure

A prerequisite for the testing is the availability of a document that describes the computer system correctly and completely. This is usually one of the following documents:

- System specification
- System manual
- User manual

The correctness and completeness of the suitable document must be proven by means of the execution of all functions at the terminal. The document must be updated if necessary.

The updated document is the basis for the Test Plan and has to be checked and signed by a second person.

continued on next page

Figure 6.1 continued

< Name of the Company>
Standard Operating Procedure TEST/001

Retrospective Testing of Computer Systems
Valid from: 01.01.93   Version 2.2   Page 4 of 6

2.1 GXP Analysis

The document selected for the test plan must be examined according to the GXP relevance of its functions. GXP relevance is based on the following critical factors:

- The function has influence on the pharmaceutical technical quality.

- The function affects medical drug safety.

- The function has influence on the data that become part of the registration documentation.

- The function is critical because of another important reason.

If one of these questions is answered in the positive, then the considered function is GXP relevant. If a function is not seen as GXP relevant, this must be justified in writing. During GXP analysis the following marks will be fixed in the text using a text marker:

- *Green:* the function is not GXP relevant.

- *Blue:* the function is GXP relevant and must be tested.

- *Yellow:* the function is indeed GXP relevant, but is based directly on the functionality of the underlying and widespread programming or operating system and therefore does not need to be tested, e.g., primary fields in a database system.

- *Pink:* the test is already covered by other test cases.

continued on next page

Figure 6.1 continued

<Name of the Company>
Standard Operating Procedure No. TEST/001

Retrospective Testing of Computer Systems
Valid from: 01.01.93   Version 2.2   Page 5 of 6

2.2 Test Plan Development

For the blue marked functions a Test Plan must be developed. For this purpose the blue marked text will be given a consecutive number and will be transmitted with this number into a new document, the Test Plan. Thus, the selected part of the document becomes a Test Case.

Thereafter, the test goals will be derived from the Test Case and written under the test case. The test goals verbally describe what should be proven. For each test goal a test procedure must be developed that describes the test and its flow in detail. The following items should be considered:

- Definition of suitable test data

- Description of the test execution

- Formulation of the expected results

- Description of the documentation method used

Thus, the finished test plan has the following structure:

```
test case 1
    test goal 1
        test procedure 1
            test data 1
            test execution 1
            expected results 1
            documentation method 1
        test procedure n
    test goal n
test case n
```

The test plan must be approved and signed by a second competent person.

continued on next page

Figure 6.1 continued

< Name of the Company>
Standard Operating Procedure TEST/001

Retrospective Testing of Computer Systems

Valid from: 01.01.93   Version 2.2   Page 6 of 6

2.3 *Test Execution and Documentation*

The tests must be executed and documented as described in the Test Plan. If technically possible and meaningful, a regression testing tool should be used in order to support ongoing evaluations.

The test results must be compared to the expected results and the conformity must be reported and signed by a second competent person.

If the test goal cannot be reached, the computer system must be modified according to the SOP *Error Handling and Correction*. The tests must be repeated until all test goals are met.

3 Distribution

(company specific)

4 Appendices

None

Figure 6.2: Relevant Part of the LIMS User Manual

	LIMS User Manual	
Version 3.4	Released 01.05.92	Page 45 of 198

Chapter 5. Manual Input of Analytical Results

After choosing menu item *Manual input of analytical results* from the main menu, the following screen appears:

Sample Number: ____

Product Number: _____ Product Name: _____
Lot-No. _____

After input of the sample number, which is taken from the analytical control form, the fields in the second row of the screen will be filled with the corresponding product number, product name, and Lot-No. Thereafter, the second part of the screen mask appears, which serves for the input of the analytical results and for the control against the limits:

Sample Number: 1234
Product Number: PRCK   Product Name: ISOBAL Tabl.
Lot-No. E555

Parameter	Value	Unit	Lower Limit	Upper Limit
Hardness	_____	N	50.0	80.0
Friability	_____	%	0.1	0.3
Weight	_____	mg	475	525

After the input of each result, the LIMS compares the value against the limits and gives the following error message, if the value is outside the limits:

"Value is outside the limits, correct with <C> or abort with <A>"

Figure 6.3: Test Cases Derived from the User Manual

Test Case 1: It must be proven that after selecting the menu item *Manual input of analytical results* from the main menu, the expected screen does in fact appear complete with all the fields described in the User Manual.

Test Case 2: It must be proven that after the input of a valid sample number, the corresponding product number, product name, and lot-no. will be displayed. For this purpose a sample must first be set up.

Test Case 3: It must be proven that the correct parameters with the corresponding units of measurements and the limits appear on the screen. For this purpose, a product specification must be set up first.

Test Case 4: It must be proven that the analytical values are checked correctly against the limits.

Test Case 5: It must be proven that after the appearance of the error message, the processing can be continued as specified (with <C> or <A>).

Figure 6.4: Test Goals Developed from Test Case 4

Test Goal 1: It must be proven that an analytical value within the limits is accepted by the system without the error message.

Test Goal 2: It must be proven that the error message appears if the analytical value is below the lower limit.

Test Goal 3: It must be proven that the error message appears if the analytical value is above the upper limit.

Figure 6.5: Test Instructions for Test Goal 2

Test Instruction 1

test data: The test data will be derived from ISOBAL Tablets, Lot-No. E555

test execution: After the selection of the parameter screen for lot-no. E555, the value *49,9* for the parameter *Hardness* must be typed in, followed by <CR>.

expected result: The following error message appears: "Value is outside the limits, correct with <C> or abort with <A>."

test documentation method: A screen copy is made after the appearance of the error message.

Figure 6.6: Test Documentation

Test Documentation for LIMS

Test case 4	Test goal 2	Test instruction 1

Test evaluation: The test result corresponds to the expected result

Tested by: Franz Maier   date: 05.09.93   Signature: _____

Approved by: Heinz Kunze   date: 07.09.93   Signature: _____

Test documentation:

Sample Number: 1234
Product Number: PRCK   Product Name: ISOBAL Tabl.
Lot-No. E555

Parameter	Value	Unit	Lower Limit	Upper Limit
Hardness	_____	N	50.0	80.0
Friability	_____	%	0.1	0.3
Weight	_____	mg	475	525

Value is outside the limits, correct with <c> or abort with <A>

REFERENCES

1. R. F. Tetzlaff, *GMP Documentation Requirements for Automated Systems:* Part III, FDA Inspections of Computerized Laboratory Systems (Pharmaceutical Technology International, October 1992).

2. A. J. Trill, *Computerized Systems and GMP—A UK Perspective:* Part II, Inspection Findings (Pharmaceutical Technology International, March 1993).

3. The Red Apple Document, *Computerized Data Systems for Nonclinical Safety Assessment—Current Concepts and Quality Assurance* (Drug Information Association, Maple Glenn, USA, 1988).

4. A. J. Trill, *Computerized Systems and GMP—A UK Perspective:* Part III, Best Practices and Topical Issues (Pharmaceutical Technology International, May 1993).

5. PMA–CSVC, "Validation Concepts for Computer Systems Used in the Manufacture of Drug Products," (Pharmaceutical Technology, May 1986).

6. G. J. Myers, *The Art of Software Testing* (John Wiley & Sons, New York, 1979).

7

Data Center Management and Good Practices

Dr. Heinrich Hambloch
European Consultant, Systems Validation
GITP: Good Information Technology Practices
Hofheim, Germany

The management of a departmental computer center in a pharmaceutical environment influences the overall quality and thus the validation status of the applications used there. Before providing a detailed introduction of the steps necessary for the operation of a computer center under GXP conditions (X traditionally refers to C, L, and M here), all factors which can influence the validation status of an application are to be considered. Figure 7.1 shows the six factors, together with those organizations usually responsible for the quality of these factors.

The first two factors, the quality of hardware and system software, are determined by the manufacturer of these systems and cannot be influenced by the pharmaceutical entrepreneur. If completely configured application software is acquired, this can also be applied to the factors three (application kernel) and four (configured application).

With the factors five and six—the environmental conditions for the hardware and the management of the computer center—the pharmaceutical entrepreneur can influence the quality of the application. This is because the computer center is normally managed by him, with his employees and in his buildings.

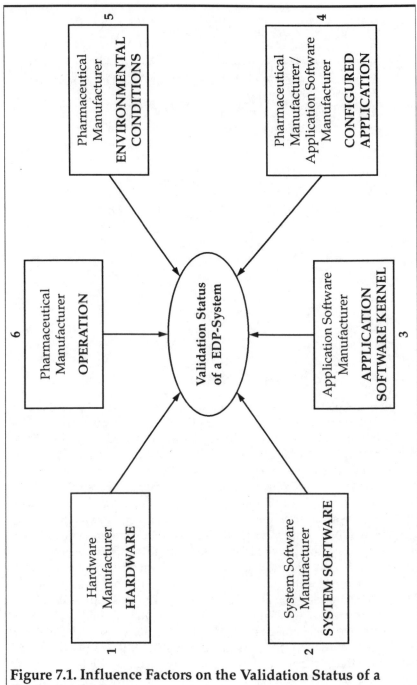

Figure 7.1. Influence Factors on the Validation Status of a Computer System

This chapter presents a system of SOPs and printed forms that have been proven by industry experience. They are applied to the operation of a computer center and show how a computer center can be operated in a GXP environment.

THE PRINCIPLE OF SOPs AND FORMS IN THE PHARMACEUTICAL INDUSTRY

Working with SOPs and forms has been practiced for a long time in the pharmaceutical industry. SOPs serve to describe operational details exactly in order to guarantee their correct realization and to allow for their control. Examples are as follows:

- Calibration instructions for analytical instruments.

- Cleaning prescriptions for devices and rooms.

- Instructions for protective clothes.

The advantages of SOPs are obvious:

- The same task is done the same way everywhere.

- Work is done correctly and completely and nothing is omitted.

- New employees are trained faster.

To complete the SOPs, printed forms are used to record work results. It is certified by signature that the work has been done according to the directives of the SOP. Therefore, the system of SOPs allows for back-checking at any time to see

- According to which procedure a work has been done.

- Who has done it, when it was done, and with what result.

This ensures a complete documentation of the development or production of a drug. Additionally, sources of error can be found and eliminated more easily by means of the SOP documented procedure. This can contribute to higher quality for a process over time.

APPLICATION OF SOPs AND FORMS TO COMPUTER SYSTEMS

Whereas the system of SOPs and forms has been common practice in the traditional work of the pharmaceutical development and production for decades, it is relatively new in the use of computer systems in pharmaceutical companies. This is true, despite the fact that data processing has become more and more important for the development and production of a drug product. It can even be said today that modern drug development and production is almost impossible without data processing. Computer systems have increasingly made their entry during the last 15 years, and their safe operation has not been consciously addressed.

There was the common opinion that hardware and software held a kind of automatic and self-evident intrinsic quality with no need for special care. No pharmaceutical entrepreneur could imagine taking an autoclave into operation without preliminary qualification and validation. Hardware and software, however, have often been used without further examination, even recently, with blind confidence in the developers and methods of this wonderful technology.

Ten years ago this circumstance was first taken into account by means of directives by the authorities (1). These directives require that data processing systems as part of the pharmaceutical development and production process are to be treated like traditional pharmaceutical devices and procedures. Consequently, they are to be validated.

The directives, however, do not prescribe exactly how these computer systems are to be validated. They do not explain which SOPs and which forms with what contents must exist and must be followed.

Later in this chapter a set of SOPs and forms with proforma contents in keywords is presented for the operation of a typical departmental computer center. These SOPs and their contents are the result of the author's many years of experience as the manager of a pharmaceutical computer center in the quality assurance department. They also include his experiences as a validation consultant.

In consulting work, the experience has been that SOPs with the same title differ considerably from company to company. Therefore, it is of no use presenting completed SOPs here (except for one as an example). They can be applied only in few cases. It is rather a presentation of the cornerstones of these SOPs that should be taken into consideration during implementation. How they are converted optimally within a company can only be usefully worked out in a consulting process, taking the whole environment into consideration.

A TYPICAL DEPARTMENTAL COMPUTER CENTER

A typical computer center in a pharmaceutical company is represented in the following discussion. Such computer centers are found in research and development departments such as toxicology or galenical, in production departments such as inventory administration, and in quality control laboratories. The SOPs described are written for use in this typical department computer center.

Such a computer center typically consists of the following:

- A midrange departmental computer

- Storage media such as hard disks and tape drives

- Connected PCs and terminals

- Printers

- Data connections to the outer world

Figure 7.2 shows a schematic overview of such a computer center and the connection of its individual components. What follows next is a description of those SOPs that ensure the secure operation of such a typical center.

SOPs FOR THE OPERATION OF A DEPARTMENT COMPUTER CENTER

Principles

Before the details of everyday operation are described for a computer center, one should put down on a paper the principles according to which the computer center should be operated and which SOPs are necessary for it. This chapter is like a table of contents for all SOPs.

To ensure that this chapter does not keep hanging in a vacuum, it should be defined in the Validation Master Plan of the company as the basic document for every internal computer center. The SOPs for the operation of a pharmaceutical computer center are, as a consequence, integrated into the internal SOP-outline of the company according to Figure 7.3.

Some ideas for the contents are specified here in keywords. The first suitable component from the point of view of clearness is a short description of the tasks of the computer center. After that, all the SOPs that are necessary for the operation of the computer center are specified:

- Determination of the SOP structure

- Description of the responsibilities

- Change control and system description for hardware

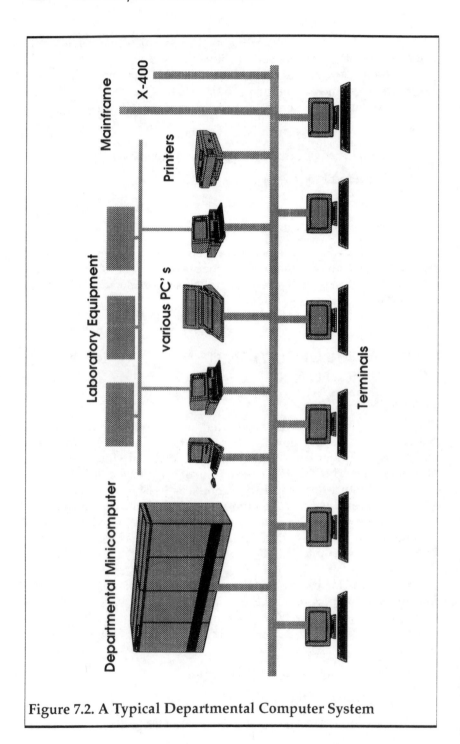

Figure 7.2. A Typical Departmental Computer System

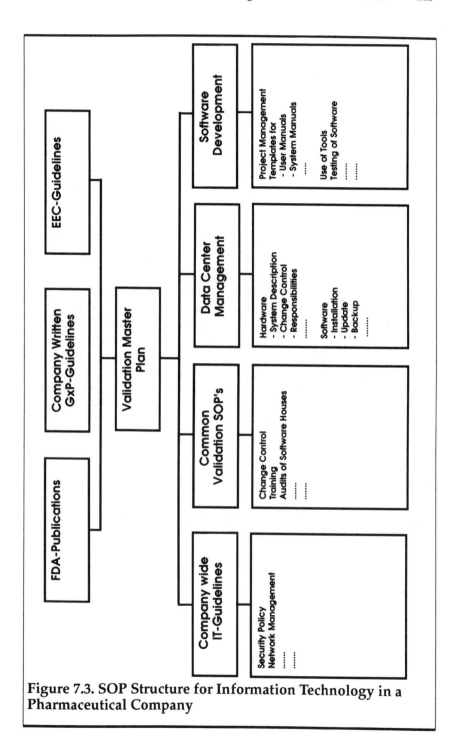

Figure 7.3. SOP Structure for Information Technology in a Pharmaceutical Company

- Preventive maintenance

- Prevention, detection, and correction of errors

- System boot and shutdown

- Control of environmental conditions

- Contingency plans and emergency operation

- Backup and restore

- Security

- Installation and update of purchased system software

- Development and change control system software procedures

Furthermore, there should be described the directives and official guidelines that are decisive for the contents of the SOPs (e.g., EEC addendum "Computerized Systems" for the GMP field or the GALP guidelines of the U.S. EPA for the GLP field (Draft) or a mixture of both, etc.). It should be clearly expressed that the SOP producer is also responsible for its implementation (i.e., he/she has to keep up-to-date in this special field).

If not yet described in other company SOPs, the management of SOPs (the procedure of modification of SOPs or putting them into operation) can be determined here.

Determination of the SOP Structure

To facilitate the adherence to the working process described in the SOP, a uniform structure for all SOPs is most successful. The following basic structure has proven useful in practice and should also be described in the form of an SOP:

- Page 1: Signatures

- Page 2: Table of contents

- Chapter 1: General

- Chapter 1.1: Purpose

- Chapter 1.2: Principles

- Chapter 1.3: Validity

- Chapter 2: Procedure description

- Chapter 3: Distribution list

- Chapter 4: Enclosures

According to the company other items can be added, for example, the archive place or references to special literature. Most important is that a homogenious and clear structure be established. Poorly structured SOPs are difficult to understand and hard to follow.

On every page of the SOP there should be a heading including the following indications:

<Name of the company>
Standard Operating Procedure for computer center <name> <SOP no.>
<SOP title>
version <number>   valid from:<date>   page <n> of <N>

The indications in square brackets are to be entered according to the SOP.

Page 1: Signatures

The following persons should sign here:

- The author, certifying the contents to be correct and complete.

- A second person (colleague or manager), for the examination of the correctness and completeness of the contents.

- The person responsible for the GXP, for conformity with authority guidelines, and for the SOPs conformity to the internal requirements of the company.

- The person who releases the SOP.

Page 2: Table of Contents

It has proven to be appropriate to use not more than four hierarchies per chapter for the assignment of numbers. The assignment of numbers is suitably made in arabic format.

Chapter 1: General.

Chapter 1.1: Purpose. This chapter points out which procedure is described by the SOP.

Chapter 1.2: Principles. The superior directives, prescriptions, common practices and so on that make this SOP necessary are described.

Chapter 1.3: Validity. Persons or departments who have to perform according to the SOP are specified here. Persons are referred to by their position (e.g., system manager), not by their names.

Chapter 2: Description of the procedure. Here a detailed procedure is described to perform the work. This is the real kernel of the SOP.

Chapter 3: Distribution list. The distribution list specifies those persons who receive the SOP and all the updates.

Chapter 4: Enclosure. All enclosures, such as program procedures or graphics (e.g., hardware diagrams) are put together here in the SOP.

The SOP should be written by the person with the best know-how. Normally, these are the system managers and the operators of the computer center. More difficult is the control by the person responsible for GXP. This person normally does not have the necessary computing experience to judge how well the directive conforms to regulations. Therefore, it is recommended to assign to the GXP position a person who has both pharmaceutical and data processing know-how.

Description of the Responsibilities

Purpose: This SOP determines the responsibilities for all GXP relevant work being done in the computer center.

Contents: An organigram is useful. Each job specified in it should be described in detail. This can be realized in this SOP or be part of the job description of the specific person.

As an example, a description of the tasks and responsibilities of an operator II is specified here.

- Control of the backup logfiles according to the "Backup" SOP

- Daily control of the error logfiles according to the SOP *Prevention, detection, and correction of errors*

- Implementation of new user accounts according to the SOP *Security*

- Realization of the remote diagnosis according to the SOP *Preventive maintenance*

- Daily control of the environmental conditions according to the SOP *Control of the environmental conditions*

It becomes clearly visible that gerenic SOPs created in advance cannot be a great help: The division of work and the responsibilities when operating a computer center differ considerably from one company to the next, and even within one company from one center to the next.

Change Control and System Description for Hardware

Purpose: This SOP determines what procedure is to be followed for changes in the hardware components of the computer center and how the hardware documentation is kept up-to-date. The description of the hardware itself, preferably in graphics, is an enclosure of this SOP.

Contents: Due to the considerable range of effects a change of the hardware can have on a GXP environment, a graduated procedure is necessary. As a consequence the SOP should separate and clearly define all cases requiring only a simple function test from the really expensive and critical changes (e.g., exchange of a printer of equal value vs. exchange of all hard disks).

The mere documentation part of changing procedure in companies is in most cases provided for, because hardware changes and extensions are realized according to an established scheme due to its commercial aspects. The investment amount for the change is budgeted for the next business year. The components are then specifically requested in the following year and usually must pass through several controlling committees. For this approval process there exist printed forms on which the changes must be justified.

From this point of view the changes are already sufficiently documented so that copies of these documents can just be added to the GXP system documentation. The permission is followed by the order placed by the purchase department of the pharmaceutical firm.

Some purchase departments carry out price comparisons between the different offers, which from an economic point of view is undoubtedly appropriate. As economic considerations can at most be secondary in a GXP environment, the utmost caution is advised.

Of primary interest is the high quality of the components (i.e., they should have been produced according to a recognized QS-system, preferably ISO 9000). This is now the case with leading hardware suppliers. Therefore, it is recommended to enter a corresponding passage concerning quality into the SOP to make quality aspects obligatory also for the purchase department.

After the components are delivered, they have to be compared with the indications in the order form. The SOP should prescribe that correctness and completeness be confirmed by signature. After a simple exchange of the same or an equal component, a function control will be sufficient. In the case of a printer, for example, the printing of a known report or in the case of a terminal the display of an input mask and the corresponding filling of the fields will be sufficient.

These function controls should be described in the SOP for the usual components of a hardware installation. Additionally, the user must be informed of the fact that even the slightest irregularities in the operation of the new device should be communicated to system management.

In case of a major change, such as the exchange of complete hard disk units on which Raw Data are stored, the SOP should prescribe that an installation and test plan including each detail of the change as well as the following tests must be developed. The correctness of this plan should be controlled by a second competent person.

The change in the system description should be documented after the plan is accomplished. The SOP should define clearly the person responsible. An exact documentation can, of course, only work if the person responsible for it knows that something has been changed. The SOP should describe that each arrival of system components be handled by this person or that this person is regularly informed about changes.

In particular, changes in the network should be approved by this person. Above all, this is important if the changes are managed centrally, as in many companies and possibly by departments that have not been working according to SOPs.

Furthermore it is recommended to discuss the documentation of external service work with the technician immediately after it is performed. The technician should document his/her work on a form that corresponds to the standard of the company's own documentation.

Preventive Maintenance

As maintenance in a computer center can be very complex, a section in several subordinate SOPs is recommended.

Purpose: This SOP describes the measures that must be taken for the preventive maintenance of the hardware components in the computer center.

Contents: Preventive maintenance in a computer center is composed of tasks performed internally and externally. One of the internal tasks is the cleaning of the computer center as well as of the easily accessible hardware components, such as the regular cleaning of magnetic tape heads.

In the introduction it was mentioned that printed forms can support the ease of work practice under an SOP. This is, of course, applicable here. For each cleaning operation a separate form should be provided. On these forms the work can be recorded according to the GXP principles and filed after they have been signed and dated.

Many of these maintenance activities are described in the manuals of the hardware manufacturer so that the SOP can refer to them directly. However, there are cases in which several activities described in the manuals have to be summarized and/or adapted for the respective installation—steady and safe working according to the original documentation is no longer guaranteed. These activities should then be summed up in the SOP.

An example for this is remote diagnosis. In this case the hardware manufacturer logs into the departmental computer and controls the contents of specific error logfiles in which errors have been recorded by the system. The service then decides whether the error rate is in the normal range or whether parts must be exchanged.

In this example, the operating system, modem, telephone system, and security are all working together and are summarized appropriately by an SOP in which all manipulations and adjustments are precisely described.

Prevention, Detection, and Correction of Errors

Purpose: This SOP describes the measures to prevent, detect, and correct errors in a computer center.

Contents: Unlike PCs, the system technology of midrange computers has operating systems that facilitate preventing, detecting, and correcting errors. It should be self-evident that in a GXP environment a company should make extensive use of these integrated tools. In addition, very intelligent error prevention utilities are offered by both operating system manufacturers and by third-party suppliers.

As a standard, error logging should be activated. In doing so the system continually writes the errors it has detected into a file. Usually the system manager can set parameters for the kind of errors that are to be entered. The logfile should be controlled at least once a day, and the SOP should clearly determine how many errors of a certain kind should lead to specific remedial measures.

An example for this is the number of correctable errors in the main memory of the computer. From a certain accumulation grade on, which is naturally system specific, service measures would be carried out, which should be described in the SOP. Such contingency limits can only be determined on the basis of daily work with the computer system and by close contact with the system manufacturer. This is another example of why it is hard to exchange SOPs between different installations.

An example for the opposite, uncritical end of the scale is a stalled printer queue. In this case a simple new start of the queue and a command to the user to print the file once more is sufficient.

As previously mentioned, in addition to these installed, simple controlling systems, there are systems that are considerably more intelligent. Such tools are programmable and can even localize errors on a graphic screen showing the overall sytem. The latter is especially interesting for network control. For example, one of these systems is able to discover that a plug of the data line has been disconnected from a terminal. The location of the terminal within the overall system is immediately shown on the screen.

Another example is the control of the hard disk filling grade. Therefore, the following can be defined in very simple language:

"When disk X is 95% full, send a mail to the system manager."

Besides these measures of avoiding and detecting errors, the elimination of errors should also be defined in the SOP (i.e., who is responsible for the correction of which kind of errors). For example, the network of the whole company is usually controlled by a central department that consequently is also responsible for the elimination of network errors. As previously mentioned, it is recommended that training in GXP and SOP concepts be given to these departments to ensure a common course and documentation of error handling.

Furthermore, it should be defined in the SOP how the users are informed in case of errors and whose task it is to inform them. In this respect, the range extends from the slow-reacting electronic mail of the office information system to an immediate logging out.

For critical systems that have a considerable influence on the GXP environment, escalation procedures should be described that can lead even to an immediate turning off of the system. This can be necessary, for example, if the situation occurs where a stockroom system that controls release or quarantine of drug raw products gets out of control due to hardware errors.

All activities during detection and elimination of errors should be documented. Here again, a form proves to be helpful. This form should record at least the following information:

- Who detected the error and when?

- Classify type of consequences—are they GXP affected or not?

- Which measures have been taken and when?

- Who eliminated the error, checked the correct function, and when was it done?

Furthermore, the SOP should prescribe that these forms are subject to periodic reviews in order to detect possible hidden long-term effects.

System Boot and Shutdown

Purpose: This SOP describes the boot and shutdown of the system as well as the order of turning on and off the power to all hardware components of the system.

Contents: In a midrange computer system, as it is defined here, situations can arise in which the system must be either shut down or even switched off. As practice shows, this is not a trivial process and should, therefore, be described in a SOP.

First, the SOP should determine who is authorized to carry out this process. Furthermore, it should be described with which commands or procedures the system is shut down and afterwards booted again. These procedures should be treated as other software is treated. That is, they must be documented, be subject to the Change Control as well as to the version handling of the software, and be checked by a second competent person.

These procedures usually include options such as a waiting period for users to log out or the indication of the disk from which the system is to be booted again. These indications must also be a part of the SOP.

When turning on or off the electric current, attention should be payed to the order in which this occurs. For example, client systems get their operating system from a server system, which, of course, has to be switched on first. The same is generally applicable for communication devices, which also boot from a server system.

Control of the Environmental Conditions

Purpose: This SOP describes the control of the environmental conditions of the computer center.

Contents: As Figure 7.1 shows, the environmental conditions are one of the six factors influencing the quality of a computer system.

The following influences are included under the environmental conditions in this context:

- Stroke of lightning

- Vibrations

- Electrostatic situation

- Temperature

- Humidity

- Fire

- Power supply

- Particulate contamination

These factors should be taken into consideration when planning a computer center. The SOP should describe how to control the really controllable influencing factors.

It is difficult to routinely measure influencing factors, such as vibrations, strokes of lightning, and electrostatic charges. In this respect, only careful planning of the location or the installation of lightning conductors and antistatic mats can help. The other factors, however, can be continually controlled with the corresponding control devices.

As far as temperature and humidity are concerned, the installation of the respective measuring devices with an alarm is recommended. The alarm is triggered if conditions exceed or fall short of the adjusted limiting values. In addition, the automatic recording of these parameters is suitable to recognize trends over time and to prevent them.

In the SOP it should be determined who reviews these records and how often, which limiting values are valid for parameters, and which measures have to be taken in case operations get out of control range. When determining the limit values, one should check with the indications of the hardware supplier to select the most sensible component and add a safety margin.

To recognize fires at an early stage, smoke detectors should be installed and checked regularly. The SOP determines the frequency and the test methodology. Additionally, hardware producers offer mini fire-fighting equipment that is installed on the individual boards in the computer and which at the slightest formation of smoke immediately spray extinguishing medium directly onto the board.

A homogeneous power supply is obtained by voltage stabilizers that are also available in combination with standby power generators. The SOP should prescribe the control of these devices.

Particulate contamination can be minimized by air conditioning filters and regular cleaning of the computer room. The frequency of these measures depends on the environment and should be described in the SOP.

Contingency Plans and Emergency Operation

Purpose: This SOP describes how work is continued after a total failure of the system for a prolonged period of time.

Contents: Before writing an SOP for Contingency Plans and Emergency Operation, one should give careful thought to the question of whether this is really necessary or if one can get along without the computer center for several days. If one decides to have an emergency operation, there are basically two possibilities:

1. Copy all backups to another computer center and to maintain the operation on a more or less provisional basis. This can be a computer center owned by the company. It can be a commercial backup computer center, or a container with a complete computer center delivered at short notice by the hardware producer.

2. Maintain the operation with a manual procedure.

If it has been decided to use a backup computer center, this SOP will certainly be one of the most extensive of the collection, because in this case a new system must be described. As an example, the rented computer center will never look like the company one. The distribution of raw data may require modification due to different disk sizes.

For a really effective operation the Disaster Recovery Plan must be practiced regularly. The safest procedure for this solution is to compare all SOPs for the operation of the company computer center critically with the system environment of the backup computer center and then to adapt it. Because of high costs, one can find such an emergency strategy only in exceptional circumstances, such as for really critical fields as with data systems in the recording and treatment of adverse drug reactions.

In most cases, however, the possibility remains to maintain a manual emergency operation. In case of the failure of a LIMS computer center, certificates of analysis could be written as formerly with a text system. Modern analytical instruments have their own computers, they can calculate the results on their own, and no longer depend on the central LIMS computer. All of these modified courses should be described precisely in the SOP and practiced regularly.

Backup and Restore

Purpose: This SOP describes backup and restore procedures for system and user data.

Contents: The SOP is divided into the subsections Backup and Restore. The respective procedures are recorded as enclosures to the SOP.

In the Backup there is a differentiation between system data and user data. System data do not change as frequently as do user data.

Different procedures are usually necessary for the system backup according to the hardware manufacturer.

In the SOP the following facts should be determined:

- How often is data backed up?

- On which media is data backed up?

- What are the names of the procedures with the backup commands?

- How many generations of tapes are stored?

- For how long is the backup data stored?

If tapes are used, the length of storage time has an affect on the quality of the stored data. After 1 year, there can be irregularities of magnetization, which requires recopying the tapes every year. The procedure required for this should be described here.

Furthermore, the SOP should determine

- How the data media are numerated

- How data are stored and where

- How defect data media are clearly marked as such and destroyed

After each data backup the logfiles should be checked for errors. For the documentation of this activity as well as for the whole data backup procedure, a form is appropriate with the following indications:

- Number of the backed up fixed disk

- Number of the backup data medium

- Date backup is performed

- Backup performed by _____ (signature)

- Logfile controlled by _____ (signature)

- Remark field for noting errors and subsequent actions

Furthermore, it should be determined what is to be done in case of errors. On magnetic tapes it often happens that, due to bad passages on the tape, whole blocks have to be left out. The SOP should, therefore, determine how many of such bad passages would disqualify a tape from being used. A reasonable decision for this can only be made after considering the history. Therefore, a periodic review of these forms is useful.

To restore the backed-up data, one should differentiate between procedures that

- Copy back a specific file.
- Copy back a whole directory, perhaps with subdirectories.
- Copy back the data of a whole disk.

Additionally, it can be necessary, according to the installation, not only to restore data exported from databases, but also to import them into the database. This should be described in the SOP.

Some operating systems allow a verification of backed-up data by reading the backup medium and comparing it with the original. This option should be prescribed in the SOP, especially for the protection of critical data such as raw data. As an alternative, there are checksum procedures that are performed (e.g., after having read every tenth block, making reports in case of errors).

Figure 7.4 (beginning on page 135) shows a complete SOP for backup and restore.

Security

Purpose: This SOP describes the security measures for the computer center.

Contents: This SOP should be divided in two chapters:

- Physical security of admission
- Software-controlled security of the system

As far as physical admission is concerned, the SOP should control which persons have admission to the computer center and when, who has the responsibility of determining this, and how this is documented. An ideal solution would be electronic door opening systems with magnetic cards that record each admission to and each exit from the computer center.

With reference to software-controlled security, the following should be determined by the SOP:

- Which user has which privileges and who determines this?
- How often do the passwords have to be changed?
- How long are the passwords?
- How are the user times determined?

Critical accounts with many privileges should always be protected with two passwords. Seldom-used accounts having many privileges should be blocked and opened only for the duration of use. This is to be documented.

Modern operating systems offer the possibility of detecting intrusions over the different possible channels. It is possible, for example, after three fruitless Log-in trials on a terminal to block this terminal for 30 minutes. Another control possibility is the detection of unauthorized access trials to data. The SOP should prescribe that such options have to be used and that the respective records have to be controlled and signed regularly.

Installation and Update of Purchased System Software

Purpose: This SOP describes the procedure of installation and update of purchased system software.

Contents: In contrast with the internally developed system programs discussed under *Development and Update of System Software Procedures*, this refers to software that serves exclusively for the operation of the system and is purchased ready-to-use. This includes, among other things, the operating system itself with all its additional programs, such as network management or safety management software.

System software is the basis for the operation of the application software. For this reason it also includes database systems because they make the implementation of application programs possible.

The SOP should determine the following:

- Preceding the installation, a backup of the old system is to be made for safety reasons.

- The installation must be performed according to a written instruction (as usually included).

- Included test programs are to be carried out.

- The new installation is to be released formally.

- The installation should be simultaneously recorded on a printer in order to document its correct performance.

The degree to which a new version is validated by company test cases depends primarily on the extent of the use of the software. If a system is used widely throughout the industry, with hundreds or thousands of installations, the large number guarantees that errors are detected quickly and eliminated by the manufacturer. This procedure is safer than a validation by the pharmaceutical entrepreneur which is, for practical purposes, impossible. Nevertheless, it is recommended to wait awhile after the publication of a new version until possible errors have been eliminated by the manufacturer.

Development and Update of System Software Procedures

Purpose: This SOP describes the procedure of creation, documentation, and modification of system software procedures.

Contents: Basically a Development and Change Control Procedure for system software is not different from that of application software. If such already exists, it can easily be modified for this purpose.

With reference to implementation, the SOP should cover the following items:

- Who is authorized to do this and what training should this person have?

- How is the software to be documented internally and how is the header structured?

- What conventions are applicable to the denomination of variables?

- What is the maximum length of an individual procedure without being divided in subprocedures?

- The procedure test is to be defined in a test plan.

- A second competent person should perform a code review.

- How long are old versions stored and where?

- Who puts the procedure into force?

Usually such system procedures are subject to modifications that are necessary to operate with new versions of the operating system. These changes must be performed under control. The SOP should, therefore, take the following items into consideration:

- Who is authorized to cause changes?

- The change should be justified in writing on a form.

- The changed program code should be controlled by a second competent person.

- A test plan is to be implemented.

- Who puts the changed version into force?

SUMMARY

Work performed under regulatory requirements in the pharmaceutical field has been successfully executed for decades using SOPs and corresponding control forms. In this chapter it was pointed out how this principle can be applied to the operation of a departmental computer center.

The introduction of such procedures is certainly not easy, because the decision margin of employees is restricted to a greater or lesser extent. Practice has shown that by a clear definition of the work in SOPs and by control through forms, the quality of the applications hosted in the computer center is increased. Due to this, the applications remain in a validated status for the influencing factors of "environment" and "operation."

Figure 7.4: An Example Backup SOP

< Name of the Company>
Standard Operating Procedure BACKUP/001
Backup for the Clinical Data Center Disk Drives
Valid from: 01.01.94   Version 2.2   Page 1 of 6

Prepared by:

_____ / _____ <NAME, DEPT.>
Signature   Date
(signs for correctness and completeness)

Approved by:

1._____ / _____ <NAME, DEPT.>
Signature   Date
(signs for control of correctness and completeness)

2. _____ / _____ <NAME, DEPT.>
Signature   Date
(signs for conformity with the GXP guidelines)

Released by:

_____ / _____ <NAME, DEPT.>
Signature   Date
(signs for release of SOP)

Continued on next page

Figure 7.4 continued

< Name of the Company>
Standard Operating Procedure BACKUP/001
Backup for the Clinical Data Center Disk Drives
Valid from: 01.01.94   Version 2.2   Page 2 of 6

Table of Contents

Continued on next page

Figure 7.4 continued

< Name of the Company>
Standard Operating Procedure BACKUP/001
Backup for the Clinical Data Center Disk Drives

Valid from: 01.01.94   Version 2.2   Page 3 of 6

---

1 General

1.1 Purpose

The SOP *Backup* describes the procedure for saving data from hard disks to magnetic tapes.

1.2 Principles

The published guidelines regarding the operating of a data center require the backup of data stored on hard disks. The *Red Apple Document* states: "Documentation regarding data security archival procedures would include backup procedures used in archiving databases . . . . "

The EPA GALP-Guideline (Draft) says in Chapter 7.8.1.8: "Standard Operating Procedures shall be established, but not limited to backup and recovery of data."

The EEC GMP addendum "Computerized Systems" states in paragraph 14: "Data should be backed-up at regular intervals . . . . "

1.3 Validity

This SOP is valid for the drug development computer center.

2 Procedure

2.1 Overview

2.1.1 User Disks

A full backup of the user disks will be performed every Monday night (Backup type UDfull). Incremental backups will be performed every night from Tuesday to Friday (Backup type UDincr, see Appendix 1).

2.1.2 Database Disks

All tables of the database have to be exported and then backed-up every night from Monday through Friday according to the scheme in Appendix 1 (Backup type DBfull).

Continued on next page

Figure 7.4 continued

< Name of the Company>
Standard Operating Procedure BACKUP/001
Backup for the Clinical Data Center Disk Drives
Valid from: 01.01.94   Version 2.2   Page 4 of 6

2.1.3 System Disk

The system disk must be backed-up after the installation of a new version of the operating system (Backup type SDfull).

2.1.4 Archiving

Data no longer needed on disk are archived on tape on the first Tuesday of every month (Backup Type ARmon). Unless otherwise specified by the user, these tapes are stored for 5 years and are copied on another tape every year.

2.2 Command Files

All backups must be performed using the procedures stored in the directory \system\backup. It is not allowed to type the backup command by hand. The names of the procedures are listed in Appendix 1.

All procedures use the system option *Verify*, which performs a read after write check. The backup procedures are subjected to the SOP *Development and Change Control of System Software Procedures*.

2.3 Tape Labels

The unique label for each tape is composed of the following:

- Backup type (Appendix 1)

- The number of the disk drive according to the SOP *Change Control and System Description of Hardware*

- The running number for each tape for that disk drive

- The generation number separated by dashes

Example:

Backup type: DBfull
Disk drive number: DUA1
Tape no. 3
Generation no. 2
Resulting label: DBfull-DUA1-3-2

Continued on next page

Figure 7.4 continued

< Name of the Company>
Standard Operating Procedure BACKUP/001
Backup for the Clinical Data Center Disk Drives
Valid from: 01.01.94   Version 2.2   Page 5 of 6

2.4 Marking and Separation of Defective Tapes

A tape is assumed to be defective if more than three write errors occurred during a backup. Defective tapes are marked with a red sticker *DEFECTIVE*. The tape content has to be overwritten with zeros using the system function *Erase Tape*. Thereafter, the tape will be brought to the central computer department for destruction. A new tape must be labeled accordingly and initialized with the system function *Initialize tape*.

2.5 Logfile Control

The logfile of the backup must be controlled for errors. If nonrecoverable errors occurred, the backup of nondaily backup types have to be repeated the following night. The control has to be signed on the Backup Logfile Control Form (Appendix 2).

2.6 Responsibilities

The responsibilities for performing the backup and controlling the logfiles is described in the SOP *Responsibilities*.

3 Distribution

This SOP will be distributed to all system managers and operators of the Clinical Data Center.

Continued on next page

Figure 7.4 continued

< Name of the Company>
Standard Operating Procedure BACKUP/001
Backup for the Clinical Data Center Disk Drives
Valid from: 01.01.94   Version 2.2   Page 6 of 6

4 Appendices

Appendix 1: Backup Scheme

Type	Frequency	Generations	Storage	Procedure
UDfull	7 days	4	Room 23	UDfull.com
UDincr	Mon.–Fri.	5	Room 19	UDincr.com
DBfull	Mon.–Fri.	5	Room 23	DBfull.com
SDfull	*	3	Room 19	SDfull.com
ARmon	monthly	1	Room 32	ARmon.com

* after installation of a new version of the operating system

Appendix 2: Backup Logfile Control Form

Date	Tape no.	Disk no.	Remarks/Actions	Signature

REFERENCE

1. FDA, *Guide to Inspection of Computerized Systems in Drug Processing* (The Blue Book), (Washington, DC: U.S. Government Printing Office: 1983-381-166:2001, February 1983).

8

Audit of External Software Vendors

Dr. Heinrich Hambloch
European Consultant, Systems Validation
GITP: Good Information Technology Practices
Hofheim, Germany

In the course of rationalization and cost reduction in pharmaceutical firms, more and more externally acquired software is used. So far, pharmaceutical firms have been able to determine the quality level of their internally developed software by themselves, but this is no longer possible with acquired software. The standard of quality of software developed externally is unknown to the purchaser beforehand.

A practical way to evaluate the quality level of a software house and also of its products is to conduct an audit. An audit is an inspection to find out whether the software house has implemented the required quality defined in a quality assurance system. The audit can be structured and thus carried out efficiently by means of the checklist presented in this chapter.

Audits of software houses have already been requested in the guidelines of the authorities and in publications made by their representatives. The Addendum "Computerized Systems" of the EEC GMP guideline states the following in paragraph 5:

> The software is a critical component of a computerized system. The user of such a software should take all responsible steps to ensure that it has been produced in accordance with a system of Quality Assurance.

In the *Red Apple Document* it says on page 18:

> Vendor development and verification/testing procedures may be reviewed by system developers to evaluate whether the procedures in use at the vendor's site are adequate for the development of a quality system, and whether these procedures were followed during system development and testing. (1)

In another publication an FDA inspector remarked:

> User firms may do on-site visits to evaluate how well a vendor has documented its validation of programs and to obtain an understanding of how the system(s) work. (2)

In the following it is pointed out how a pharmaceutical firm can

- Plan,
- Realize, and
- Evaluate

a quality audit in a software house.

It is assumed that the pharmaceutical firm has already ascertained that the product offered by the software house basically covers the required functions or that the software house is experienced in the development of applications on the specific field in case of new software to be written. As a consequence, the checklist presented here does not include any questions concerning the functionality of the system.

Of course, quality audits can also be applied to internal software development. In both cases, external and internal, the audit should be performed in a constructive atmosphere. Only if this is the case, will both sides gain profit from the experience.

The advantages of software produced with quality assurance are obvious for the pharmaceutical entrepreneur:

> The more quality that is implemented during the writing of a software, the less effort is necessary for the pharmaceutical firm, when the validation is made at a later stage.

THE PLANNING OF THE AUDIT

When planning an audit, the following items should be taken into consideration:

Circle of Participants on the Purchaser's Side

A delegation of three persons is recommended for this purpose:

- One employee or an external consultant with knowledge of software and hardware quality assurance.

- One employee with GXP know-how (X traditionally corresponds to L, M, C).

- One representative of the future user's side.

Circle of Participants on the Side of the Software House

In the course of the audit, the delegation of purchasers will undoubtedly be in contact with a number of employees of the software house. For reasons that will be explained in more detail later, the following persons should take part:

- A representative of the management.

- A representative of the quality assurance unit.

Delivery of the Audit Result to the Software House

Preceding the audit there should be an agreement that the possible purchaser will put the results of the audit at the disposal of the software house. First, this is fair toward the software house and secondly, deficiencies that were found can be eliminated more easily.

It stands to reason that the possible purchaser does not make the results accessible to any third party without the permission of the software house. Even if audits require a certain additional effort on the part of the software house, the software house is offered a gratuitous chance of improving its own quality and gets another opportunity for improving and strengthening the relationship between customer and supplier.

Delivery of the Questionnaire in Advance

The software house should be given sufficient opportunity to prepare for the audit. Therefore, the questionnaire should be sent in advance.

Duration of the Audit

For a general audit one day normally is sufficient. However, if in addition to general quality assurance, the quality of a specific product is to be examined, two days or a second day at a later date should be agreed upon.

THE REALIZATION OF THE AUDIT

As mentioned above, the audit should be realized by means of a questionnaire that helps to structure the audit and prevents omissions. That does not mean, however, that one should only stick to this list; if necessary, one might delve deeper into the matter.

The list is classified by four groups of questions:

- General questions concerning the software house

- Questions concerning quality assurance

- Questions concerning software development

- Questions concerning the quality of the software product of interest

The following discusses the questions with an explanation on the background of the respective question.

General Questions Concerning the Software House

How Many Employees Does the Software House Have?
What Has the Turnover Development Been in the Last Few Years?
How Long Has the Software House Been in Business?

The software house should be big and solid enough to be successful over the next few years (i.e., the firm should bring along all the financial requirements for a long-term business relationship).

How is the Software House Organized?

A clear structure in the division of tasks is the precondition for the development of a well-structured software. The management should be able to explain the structure by means of an actual organigram.

What Dimension Does the Product Portfolio Have?
How Many Employees Will Work on the Product of Interest?

The product in question should have a strategic meaning for the software house, so that the investment of the purchaser is also guaranteed on a long-term basis. The more employees that work on the product, the more likely this will be true.

Is the Software House Known in Pharmaceutical Circles?
Are There Any Customer References?

If the software house has worked with pharmaceutical customers, it is probable that the staff is familiar with the pharmaceutical requirements for validation, authority guidelines, and GXP. The purchaser should ask for a reference list and do some inquiries on a random sample from the list.

Is the Software House Able to Offer Long-Term Support?

To guarantee the investment, long-term cooperation is necessary. The purchaser should find out whether the software house considers itself more as a license vendor or as a long-term support partner. In doing so the purchaser should also ask for the kind of support (e.g., telephone support via hotline, etc.) available.

Questions Concerning Quality Assurance

Which Value is Assigned to Quality in the Software House?

This question should first be asked to the management, and then the auditors should find out the following points in discussion.

- Is the quality of the software one of the principal aims of the business?

- Is the management really committed to quality assurance or does it consider QA more as a nuisance, as red tape, or as an exaggerated demand made by the authorities?

- How is the staff made conscious of the importance of quality?

Does a Written Quality Assurance System Exist?

Enduring quality exists only when it is planned and controlled. Ideally, this is implemented through an internationally acknowledged QS-System. In this respect the ISO 9000-3 is one applicable standard, an interpretation of the ISO 9001 for the development of software. According to the author, a thorough implementation of ISO provides what in pharmaceutical circles is called validation.

How Are Complaints Dealt With?

Complaints should be collected and analyzed systematically by the quality assurance unit. An alarm system should be established that immediately informs the customers when serious deficiencies are discovered. The collection of complaints in a database is ideal. Additionally, there should be a description on how to perform and document "bug fixes" as contrasted with planned changes (Change Control).

How Are Beta-Tests Performed?

Before officially distributing new versions, the software house should perform Beta-Tests with a few selected customers. The result of these Beta-Tests should be documented. By using the software in practical operation, additional deficiencies can be discovered and repaired in the official new version.

There is also an interest on the part of the software house to perform Beta-Tests. By doing so the probability of expensive recall actions and the loss of image related with such actions can be minimized.

Are Internal Audits Conducted Regularly?

A QS-system is only efficient if its adherence is controlled. The best way of doing so is through regular internal audits. These audits should be recorded and the discovered deficiencies should be eliminated. The checks to be performed in the audit should be put down in writing.

Questions Concerning Software Development

This complex of questions is divided into the following domains:

- Staff
- Development methods
- Test methods
- Documentation

The questions are essentially oriented towards the life cycle model of the software.

Staff

Is the Staff Sufficiently Trained?

The better the technical know-how of the staff, the more likely it is that modern, high-quality software will be produced. If apprentices or temporary employees are involved in the development of a product requiring validation, their work should be checked with particular care.

Does the Staff Receive Sufficient Training?

Only sufficiently trained staff know the methods of modern software production. Each employee should also be trained in the methods of quality assurance. Both internal and external training should be documented. There should be a training plan of the current year for each employee.

On Average, How Long Do the Employees Stay with the Firm?

High turnover of personnel indicates a potential for problems in the working conditions. The employees' satisfaction with their working place is of decisive importance for their motivation and thus for the quality of their accomplished work. In addition, the auditors should pay attention to the working atmosphere among employees during the audit.

Development Methods

Are There Any Project Plans with Attributed Responsibilities and Time Schedules?

Good software development requires careful planning and review of the work. This includes putting down the responsibilities for the individual project parts in writing and assigning specific resources. The records of regular project meetings should be stored in order to prove the course of the project. Permanent delays or wrong estimates of resources show deficient planning.

Can it Be Shown That Each Employee Only Has Access to His/Her Own Parts of the Project?

It should be guaranteed that project development is protected by change control and security measures. A protected directory structure for the overall project is the precondition for access security.

Which Development Tools Are Used?

Maintainable software of high quality and reasonable price can only be obtained by using modern development tools. With respect to development, keeping up-to-date means, among other things, the application of CASE-Tools and relational databases.

Are There Any Prescriptions Concerning the Application of Programming Tools?

Standardized guidelines should exist for the application of tools. They should determine the following:

- How variables and registers are named
- How the code is optically structured (important for three GL languages)
- How error messages are configured
- How function keys are assigned uniformly
- How menus, screen masks, and reports are structured
- How HELP texts are structured
- How the directory and access structure for a project looks
- Which program libraries must be used

What Does the Hardware Development Environment Look Like?

The responsibility for the administration of the hardware environment in the software house should be clearly defined. This includes written working guidelines for the operation of the development computers should exist. A description of a well-controlled and well-documented hardware environment is given in Chapter 7 of this book.

Test Methods

Are There Any Prescriptions for the Performance of Tests?

A documented test procedure should exist. It should make statements on the

- Test plan.

- Test records.

The test plan should be structured as follows:

Test case 1
    Test goal 1
        test procedure 1
            test data 1
            text execution 1
            expected results 1
            documentation method 1
        test procedure n
            . . .
            . . .
    Test goal n
        . . .
        . . .
    . . .
    . . .
    Test case n

The test records include the results of the test in a form reconstructable and understandable by a third party. A detailed description of these terms is given in Chapter 6 of this book.

Is a Test Review Carried Out by a Second Person?

A second person should review the test plan in order to determine whether the test cases cover the system specifications and the design documents. The results of this review should be documented.

Are the Tests Structured in Phases?

Tests should be structured according to the different phases of the software life cycle model. These phases are divided into the following tests:

- Module test (the test of a module)

- Integration tests (the tests of the interfaces between the modules)

- System test (the test of the overall system—the cooperation of the different modules through the interfaces and the test of the application limits. All error messages should be created here.)

- Acceptance test (the test by the users against the systems specification or within the context of a beta-test)

Are Test Tools Used?

The use of test tools facilitates the regression test: The input and output of the first test run are recorded by the test tool; in doing so the test can afterward be repeated automatically, without input by the tester. The results of the new test are automatically compared to the preceding ones and deviations are indicated.

Are the Testers Different from the Developers?

To avoid conflict of interest, the testers should not be the same persons as the developers. Preferably, they should also have different managers. It has proven to be practical for employees of the software development department to also change to the test department in a job rotation and vice versa.

Does the Software House Provide Technical Support for Validation After the Installation with the Purchaser?

Some software houses have started to offer validation help to the purchaser. So, for example, one LIMS producer provides two folders filled with test cases for each field in each mask. Another software house provides complete test data sets, which can be carried out automatically with the purchaser after installation. The test results are then compared to the expected results and possible deviations are indicated.

Pharmaceutical firms should convince software houses to offer these test helps in the future as an option, so that the validation work after installation can be minimized.

Documentation

Are There Any Prescriptions Concerning Structure and Contents of the Documents?

There should be clear descriptions of how the individual documents of the different software development phases are structured and what is included in the individual chapters. By doing so a homogeneous structure is guaranteed and the introduction of new employees is facilitated. Moreover, costs are reduced, which ultimately is also in the interest of the purchaser.

Are All Documents Signed and is There a Description of the Undersigners' Responsibility?

On each document it should be clearly defined who is responsible for the

- Contents,

- Technical examination of the contents, and

- Quality examination of the document (for compliance to SOPs).

The meaning of the signatures should be described in the prescriptions concerning structure and contents of the documents.

Is the Development Documentation Structured and Complete?

The following documents should at least be provided for a well developed software system:

- **System specification:** This describes the system from the point of view of the user (what is the system supposed to do?). Among other things, all input and output as well as all processing steps, calculations, and interfaces are specified so that a future user will understand it.

- **System design document:** This describes the system from the point of view of data processing (how should the system do it?). Among other things, data models, their translation in file or database structures, as well as screen masks and interfaces are described in detail.

- **Source code:** This includes the computer commands in a programming language or parameter settings with four GL-tools.

- **Installation handbook:** This describes the process of installation on the target computer. It should also specify the required software and hardware resources, such as operating systems, compilers, database systems, printers, and so on.

- **User handbook:** This describes the operation of the system for the user and also includes the limits of applicability.

According to the complexity of the system, further documents may be necessary. Thus, process control systems may require additional engineering plans and specifications of hardware components, such as valves and thermometers, calibration prescriptions, and cabling diagrams.

Have All Documents Been Examined by a Second Person?

To minimize design deficiencies, the systems specification and the system design document should be submitted for review by a second person.

How Are Changes in Already-Released Documents Dealt With (Change Control)?

The software house should establish a Change Control Plan for each product or project. This plan should specify, among other things:

- Who is authorized to make changes in the individual documents?

- Who is in charge of the technical control of these changes?

- Who checks the quality?

- Who implements the changes?

- Who tests the changed software and how is this done?

- Who releases the changed software for use?

A printed form with all these data facilitates the adherence to the change control plan.

Questions on the Software Product

How Long is the Product on the Market?

The longer a product is on the market, the more perfected it is likely to become when monitored by a well controlled QA program. Well-maintained software has a decreasing number of deficiencies during its life.

How Often Has the Product Been Sold?

The more frequently a product is sold, and thus used, the more likely is the discovery of deficiencies. If the producer provides a reliable handling of complaints, these deficiencies will be eliminated.

How Often Has the Product Been Revised?

Too frequent release of software changes can indicate a deficient change control procedure. Moreover, frequent release changes also cost the purchaser time and resources. Rare release changes can indicate a product in retirement. The ideal is in the middle—one or two release changes per year are certainly acceptable in most cases.

Who Uses the Product?

In this respect a reference list should be provided. The satisfaction of reference customers should be checked by random sampling from the list. If possible, a meeting with a reference customer should be arranged.

Are There Regular User Meetings?

User meetings allow for the exchange of opinions among the users and for the joint formulation of desirable changes directed to the producer. The users as a group are in a stronger position toward the software house.

Can the Source Code be Deposited in a Neutral Place?

Depositing the source code with a notary (escrow account) allows the further development of the software in the case of bankruptcy of the software house. Additionally, all the internal development tools employed should be deposited along with the source code. There are also inspectors who demand the availability of the source code.

If the Software Has to be Adjusted for the Purchaser, will a QS-System Also Be Used?

To ensure a homogeneous quality standard for all system components, the same QS-system should be used for the adjustment or configuration as for the production of the kernel.

Are Older Versions Also Maintained in Case the Purchaser Does Not Want to Install the Newest Version Immediately?

Especially for the pharmaceutical sector with its high standards of quality concerning the safety of software used, firms intentionally wait some time before installing new versions. This is simply because it is very likely that early problems are then already eliminated. Therefore, it should be determined whether the software house offers the maintenance of old versions.

Does the Software House Also Provide User Training?

The software house should provide user training, because it knows the software better in the first place, and the training will thus be more effective. The quality of the training material, however, should be examined before training begins.

The Course of the Audit

The auditors should first specify who draws up the records during the audit. The course of an audit should be divided into the following five phases:

Initial Conversation with a Software House Management Representative

First the auditors should determine whether there are any reservations about individual questions on the previously delivered questionnaire.

Then the general questions about the software house should be dealt with (first part of the questionnaire).

Explanation of the QA-System

The applied QA-system should be explained by the manager of quality assurance. At that point the questions of the second part of the questionnaire can be posed.

Examination of the QA-System and Documentation by Random Samples

Now the QA-system should be checked by random samples of one product of the software house. If the purchaser is interested in a specific product of the software house, this product should be chosen. It is recommended to ask the questions of the third part of the questionnaire by means of a concrete example. For this purpose the auditors can choose a screen mask or a specific function and retrace its documentation along its life cycle.

The auditors should have a look at all documents from the test record to the system specification and check the contents. In doing so the purchaser should also pay attention to the structure and to the comprehensiveness of the contents.

Evaluation of the Product of Interest

If the meeting serves as the evaluation of a certain product, the auditors can now ask the questions on the fourth part of the questionnaire.

Summary

Finally, the first positive as well as negative impressions should be discussed with the representative of the software house management, so that he/she can give his/her view, and open questions can be settled before the official audit report.

EVALUATION OF THE AUDIT

To draw a comparison with audits of other software houses, a half-quantitative evaluation can be obtained by assigning points and weighting each question. Every pharmaceutical firm must develop this weighting itself, according to what it considers to be important or unimportant. For reasons of an easier comparison, it is recommended to make the evaluation separately for the four groups of questions.

For the evaluation of the individual questions, the following scheme of points can be applied:

Points	Judgment for the quality of answers	Points	Judgment for the quality of documentation
0	Unsatisfactory	0	No documentation exists
1	Could be better	1	Partial documentation exists
2	Good to Excellent	2	Documentation complete

Past experience has shown that too many evaluation points make the judgment process more difficult. For this reason only three possibilities are indicated.

The comparison of total points of the software houses, however, can only serve to divide the wheat from the chaff. For deeper differentiations the auditors should rely on your common sense.

SUMMARY

The method of auditing described in this chapter should help to make software houses more familiar with pharmaceutical needs. It should also help them understand the requirements of authorities that pharmaceutical firms must obey while using information technology.

The advantage of using software with proven, assured quality is that the pharmaceutical entrepreneur only has to deal with the validation activities after installation. The software house has already covered all the preceding activities.

The advantage for the software house is that it is acknowledged as a long-term business partner of the pharmaceutical industry. Software houses not providing constant quality assurance in the future will be confronted with many difficulties in the pharmaceutical market.

It is the task of the pharmaceutical entrepreneur to intensify the idea of quality assurance in the software houses in the future. An audit is an appropriate opportunity for doing that.

REFERENCES

1. Computerized Data Systems for Nonclinical Safety Assessment—Current Concepts and Quality Assurance (*Red*

Apple Document), (Drug Information Association, Maple Glen, USA, 1988).

2. R. F. Tetzlaff, GMP Documentation Requirements for Automated Systems: Part III, *FDA Inspections of Computerized Laboratory Systems*, (Pharmaceutical Technology International, October 1992), p. 4.

9

Clinical Data Systems, GCP Validation, and CANDA

Dr. Teri Stokes
International Consultant
Pharmaceutical Business Group
Digital Equipment Corporation
Basel, Switzerland

Validation of computer systems under Good Clinical Practice (GCP) regulations is a 1990s initiative of the EC Committee on Proprietary Medicinal Products (CPMP). In contrast, GMP and GLP computer validation dates back to the FDA directives of the early 1980s. Given this time difference, one often finds that Medical Directors are less aware than their manufacturing counterparts of the priority for validation of computer systems in GCP-regulated areas.

Industry focus for this work is stronger in Europe than elsewhere due to the 1991 implementation of the new EC GCP Guideline Directives. Section 3.10 of the EC GCP states that

> The sponsor must use validated, error-free data processing programs with adequate user documentation. (1)

Various other statements throughout its chapter on data handling continue to stress the need to verify computer performance and document the integrity of clinical data handled by electronic systems used at both sponsor and investigator sites.

This new regulatory focus comes at a time when the industry is looking very closely at its clinical development processes for ways to improve its time to market for new products. Company efforts to validate clinical data systems can also be used to examine and optimize the data flow of the people and paper systems interacting with computer systems. The return on investment (ROI) for GCP validation of clinical data systems should include more than compliance to regulations. It should also contribute to optimizing the speed of data handling and assure the quality and integrity of study data used to develop the Dossier, NDA, and CANDA submissions.

BUSINESS LIFE CYCLE FOR GCP VALIDATION

Regulatory authorities are pressuring the Drugs and Devices Industry to provide documented proof (validation) of their CONTROL for the Safety, Efficacy, Quality, and Cost of new therapies. Processes and procedures that include computerized systems must be kept under CONTROL for areas of the business affecting Safety, Efficacy, and Quality of product. The new element of cost control has been introduced to help countries meet soaring healthcare costs. These pressures all have their impact on data collected during Phases I–IV of clinical trials.

The final output of the pharmaceutical research and development process is not rats, pills, or patients. The output is data, which is, hopefully, in the form of information. When the data handling process is under control, there is a "flow" of data and information. When the process is out of control, it becomes a "flood" of data and in some cases it is so out of control that companies are drowning in a "sea" of data with little or no useful information.

Corporate management in the Drugs and Devices Industry faces many global challenges and looks to go beyond just controlling the situation. Management is pressuring the organization to OPTIMIZE all processes for the Safety, Efficacy, Quality, and PROFIT of new therapies. Management looks for more than just compliance. It wants continual improvement in its business results (e.g., more profitable products to market in less time). This business life cycle for validation is shown in Figure 9.1. The GCP, GLP, GMP areas are highlighted in Figure 9.2 where GMP for trial supplies is shown in R&D and Phase IV in addition to GMP for full production in Manufacturing.

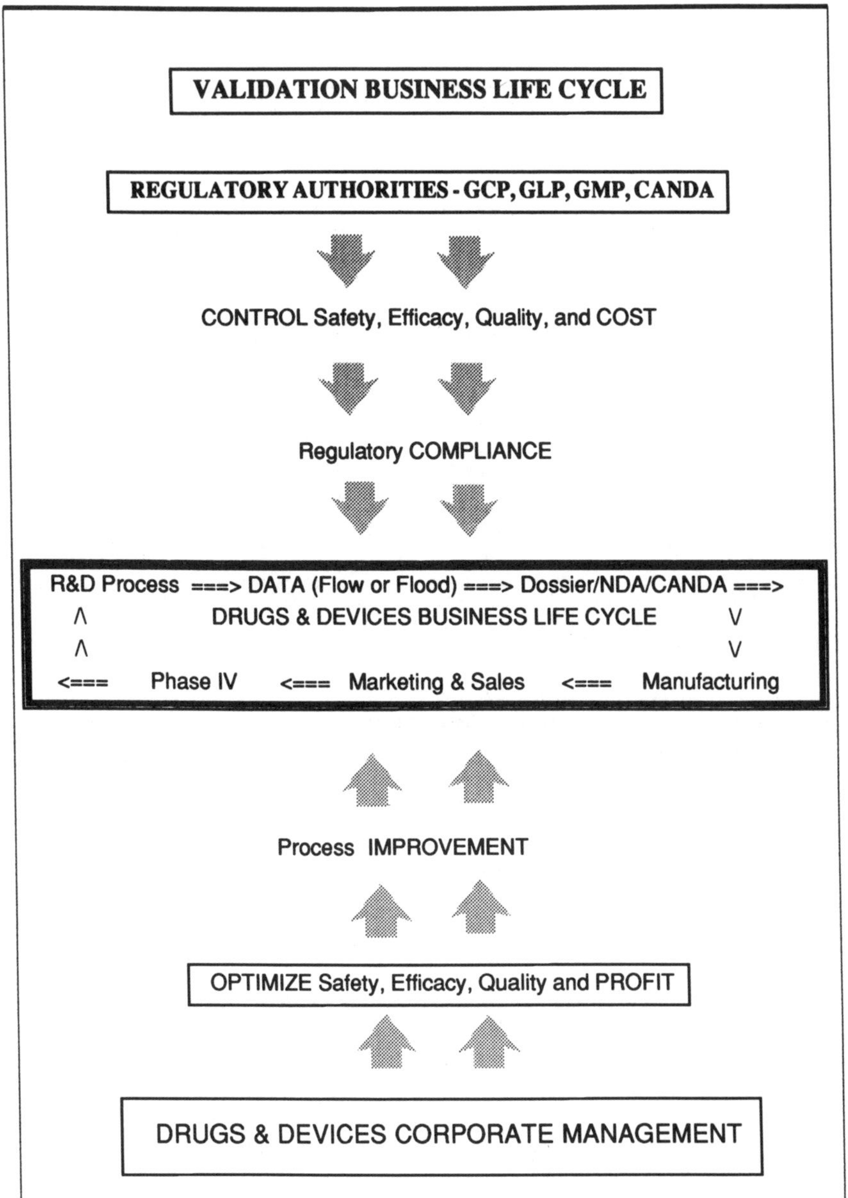

VALIDATION BUSINESS LIFE CYCLE

REGULATORY AUTHORITIES - GCP, GLP, GMP, CANDA

CONTROL Safety, Efficacy, Quality, and COST

Regulatory COMPLIANCE

R&D Process ===> DATA (Flow or Flood) ===> Dossier/NDA/CANDA ===>
  ^   DRUGS & DEVICES BUSINESS LIFE CYCLE   V
  ^   V
<===   Phase IV   <===   Marketing & Sales   <===   Manufacturing

Process IMPROVEMENT

OPTIMIZE Safety, Efficacy, Quality and PROFIT

DRUGS & DEVICES CORPORATE MANAGEMENT

Figure 9.1: Validation Life Cycle in Business

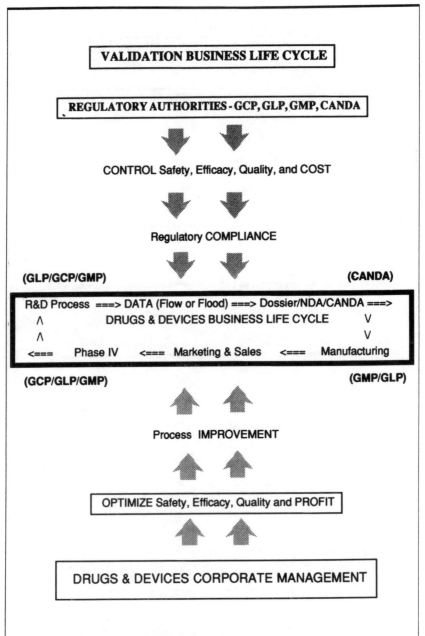

Figure 9.2: Computer Validation Areas

THE GCP DIFFERENCE FOR COMPUTERS

Data handling in the GCP domain is very people intensive and the human interface to electronic systems in this area is multidisciplinary. Use of an electronic Case Report Form (CRF) for gathering study data could have a physician, a study nurse, or a medical clerk doing data entry of trial results at the investigator site. Training for these people, user documentation, and system validation for the device on location must all be documented under EC GCP requirements.

Regional data entry by company personnel at a subsidiary location could be done by clinical research associates (CRAs), Medical Monitors, or Study Directors. Again, training, documentation, and system validation needs per site must comply with GCP. System security, authorized access control to data, and verification of communication transmissions back to central clinical databases also apply for each site doing entry of regulated data.

The software used to manage CRF data is usually reconfigured separately to meet the demands of each new study design. Both back-end database design and front-end data entry screens change for every new trial protocol. The degree of change can also be dramatic with different therapeutic areas using the same computer system. Analysis of trial results is also done with custom-coded algorithms for each study. GCP control of these dynamic software environments is posing new validation challenges for clinical computerized systems.

DATA SYSTEMS THAT ARE GCP REGULATED

Regulated data systems in the GCP area include those handling data that are intended to prove to regulatory authorities that the new therapy is safe and medically effective, that the trial drug/device was made with controlled quality, and that the new drug/device is cost-effective relative to other therapies on the market. This includes data handling for CRFs, adverse event reports (AEs), clinical lab results, toxicology and safety studies, quality testing on trial supplies, pharmacy tracking of trial drugs, subject randomization lists, automated labeling for blinded trial supplies, and so on.

Since much of the proof to authorities is based on statistical analysis of trial data, the statistical software used is a key system to include in GCP validation efforts. Section 3.15 of the EC GCP states that

> If data are transformed during processing, the transformation must be documented and the method validated. (2)

The March 1993 draft copy for review of the EC CPMP Note for Guidance on Biostatistics states the following:

11. Data entry and data verification

Data entry and verification are now generally the responsibility of data management units with their own rapidly developing rules and standard operating procedures (SOPs). The credibility of the results depend strongly on the quality and validity of methods used for data coding, entry, and plausibility checks, and of course on the quality and validity of the software for processing the data statistically. **Regular validation of software used in data management and biostatistical units is mandatory.** (3)

Bolding of the last sentence is done by the author, because it is such a clear statement of current EC thinking in this area. This is important for both EC companies and non–EC companies who want to sell drugs and devices in the European Union countries.

WHERE COMPANIES USUALLY START GCP SYSTEMS VALIDATION

Most companies begin their GCP validation efforts with their computer systems that host CRF databases. A second common priority is to validate computer systems hosting AE databases. The logic to this is apparent as the CRFs and AEs contain the primary sources of efficacy and safety data for company products. The initial validation of each of these systems is an individual project requiring a team of people from the various disciplines who work with the system. It is very much an end user effort and not solely an IT or QA function.

The third priority is to examine the statistical systems. These are most often using software from SAS, Inc. Companies find it useful to come to this area after experiencing the practical lessons of doing a major system validation. It is preferable that the statistical GCP project team have several members participating in the previous CRF or AE validation project in order to gain experience in validation approaches.

It is a serious challenge for GCP validation activities to address the individual programmer flexibility usually allowed in the SAS software environment of many biostatistics departments. Some good software engineering practices (GSEPs) will need to be agreed upon and introduced through SOPs and documented code activities for this area to operate in a validated manner. Here the human interface is extremely important to data integrity. Validation work can also provide a rich opportunity for GCP control to be combined with corporate optimization goals. Clear, well-documented statistical reports and procedures raise few questions and speed approvals at regulatory authorities.

MEMBERSHIP OF THE GCP VALIDATION TEAM

In the experience of this author, it is important that a company's own people be directly involved in all aspects of GCP systems validation. This is not an area to be handed over to an outside validation team. So much of ongoing clinical practice is interconnected with system use that the human interface itself is a part of the system and must participate in the validation.

The project needs a management mandate to commit time and resources to the validation effort. Usually the Director of Biostatistics or the Head of Clinical Data Management will be an active driver of the project and this person manages the resource mandate. It is important that the Medical Director and Corporate Quality Management participate in final review and signature approval of the GCP systems validation efforts as they have ultimate GCP compliance responsibility for the company.

A typical team for the validation of a CRF management application would be the following:

- Director of Biostatistics* *or* Head of Clinical Data Management
- Clinical QA person (to develop ongoing GCP audits)*
- Software Database System Manager (person who runs the CRF software application)*
- Hardware Platform System Manager (person who manages the hardware, network, and underlying software for the CRF software application)*
- Corporate Quality person (to do a final audit)
- Database Administrator (person who sets up files for a study)*
- Clinical Research Associate (person who collects trial CRFs)
- Study Monitor (person responsible for all trials/product)
- Statistician*
- Data Entry persons (local and remote)
- Project Manager (person outside of clinical to drive actions)*

- External experts as needed for consulting on GCP validation or specific product experience*

* = Suggested members for a Test Plan Working Group

Having a Project Manager on the team from outside the medical function helps the team keep on focus despite the inevitable ongoing emergencies of conducting clinical trials. This person's sole responsibility in Medical is the success of the validation effort. This will keep the project on track despite operational pressures.

External experts on the team are expensive and should be used carefully for the highest leverage that their expertise can bring. When product-specific software experience can save the team weeks or months in designing a useful Test Plan, then use specific software experts. If you just need more hands at the keyboard to input a Test Procedure Script, do not use them. Use more data entry clerks instead. The clerks cost you less and they have the job enrichment experience of participating in a computer validation project.

THE ROLE OF THE GCP VALIDATION TEAM & THE TEST PLAN WORKING GROUP

The role of the Validation Team is to develop a Validation Plan for the project. The Validation Plan should identify all activities required to document the validated state of the target system in compliance with GCP. In the case of a CRF Management System, this team would discuss the company's experience with the CRF Management application and would identify the following:

- Specific CRF software and supporting hardware, software and network "platform" elements to be included in the Plan
- Key areas requiring new SOPs
- Edits to job descriptions for CVs
- Training needs
- Audits of hardware, software, and service suppliers
- Cataloging of key system documents
- Development of a written history of past and present system experience
- Resources needed to implement the plan
- Resources needed for ongoing validation efforts

A special subset of the validation team, identified by (*) in the team listing on pages 163–164, would form a Test Plan Working Group. This subgroup would develop Test Plans for the CRF Software and Platform systems. They would later involve others in the effort to write Testing Procedure Scripts for specific software functions targeted by the Test Plan for active testing.

A major task for the working group is to define the limits of the system being tested so that the effort is doable. Figure 9.3 provides a list of definitions for the various activities performed in this area. (4) Figure 9.4 contains a list of items to be included in developing testing plans for computerized systems. (5) The ANSI/IEEE Std 829-1983 document provides a tutorial discussion of each of the sixteen items listed in the Test Plan Outline.

In its 1987 inspector training documents on Software Development, the U.S. FDA mentioned ANSI/IEEE and ISO standards as being useful references for assuring software quality. This author has found it practical to have Test Plan Working Groups adapt the following standards to their own situation.

- ANSI/IEEE Std 1008-1987: IEEE Standard for Software Unit Testing

- ANSI/IEEE Std 829-1983: IEEE Standard for Software Test Documentation

---

Figure 9.3: Validation and Test Definitions (Adapted from ANSI IEEE Std 729-1983)

Validation Plan—A document written to describe all roles, responsibilities, and activities surrounding the validation of a computerized system.

Test Plan—A document prescribing the approach to be taken for intended testing activities under the scope of a Validation Plan. The plan typically identifies the items to be tested, the testing to be performed, test schedules, personnel requirements, reporting requirements, evaluation criteria, and any risks requiring contingency planning.

Test Procedure Script—Document written to give detailed instructions for the setup, operation, and evaluation of results for a given test for a specific module of the target system being tested under the Test Plan.

Test Suite—A set of associated test procedure scripts combined to form a test procedures document for ongoing testing use.

Test Report—A document describing the conduct and results of the testing carried out for a system or system component.

Figure 9.4: Test Plan Outline ANSI/IEEE std 829-1983

A test plan shall have the following structure:

1. Test-plan identifier	9. Test deliverables
2. Introduction	10. Testing tasks
3. Test items	11. Environmental needs
4. Features to be tested	12. Responsibilities
5. Features not to be tested	13. Staffing and training needs
6. Approach	14. Schedule
7. Item pass/fail criteria	15. Risks and contingencies
8. Suspension criteria and resumption requirements	16. Approvals

---

- ANSI/IEEE Std 983-1986: IEEE Guide for Software Quality Assurance Planning
- ANSI/IEEE Std 730-1989: IEEE Standard for Software Quality Assurance Plans
- ISO 9000-3 Quality management and quality assurance standards—Part 3: Guidelines for the application of ISO 9001 to the development, supply, and maintenance of software

Standards documents from ANSI/IEEE are available by writing

The Institute of Electrical and Electronics Engineers, Inc.
345 East 47th Street
New York, NY 10017-2394, USA

The International Organization for Standardization (ISO) has chapters per country that can supply ISO 9000 documents and a worldwide headquarters in Geneva, Switzerland.

All of these standards are generic good software engineering practice (GSEP) guides that are applicable to aerospace software projects as well as local instrument drivers. These standards all assume full life cycle activity for software systems, making them especially useful as validation support for the development of new software in regulated environments. The Test Plan Working Group must apply some common sense to adapting them to the specific complications of an existing computerized system, such as a CRF management system.

Most CRF management systems layer on top of other software such as a relational database. In addition, they may use the security features of the hardware operating system or have close interactions with a statistical package. It is important to document the limits of testing activity and give a reason for the limits. For instance, the company may only use certain modules of a vendor's system and may then state a reliance on the vendor's QA to assure unused elements.

SOFTWARE VALIDATION PLAN FOR AN EXISTING CRF MANAGEMENT SYSTEM

This author recommends that the development of a Validation Plan begin with a workshop session for the whole Validation Team. At this session a common set of reference documents relevant to GCP and systems validation is presented to each participant and a common understanding is developed for what GCP validation of computerized systems is all about. People share their experiences about using the target system and discuss the areas they consider to be of GCP concern.

Writing the actual Validation Plan document is done by the Project Manager after inputs from the Validation Team sessions. A good standard reference for developing this document is the ANSI/IEEE Std 1012-1986. This IEEE Standard for Software Verification and Validation Plans covers all phases of the life cycle of writing a new software system and can also be easily adapted to existing and vendor-supplied systems. Figure 9.5 shows the ANSI/IEEE suggested outline of the contents of a validation plan. (6)

When one is writing a validation plan for an existing system, the active work on Test Plans is done for the Operation and Maintenance Phase only. A written historical review by internal developers is used to cover prior phases of the software life cycle for company-developed systems. Vendor-supplied documents would do the same for systems purchased commercially.

Writing a System History

When validating existing systems within the Operation and Maintenance phase of the software life cycle, the company needs to write a history of its experience with the software since its first installation. This should be done by people who have had the longest experience operating the system. The history should be supported by reference to maintenance logs and other system documents generated during the life of its use in the company. Figure 9.6 gives a checklist of activities to support this history writing effort.

Figure 9.5: Software Verification & Validation Plan Outline (ANSI/IEEE Std 1012-1986)

1. Purpose

2. Referenced Documents

3. Definitions

4. Verification & Validation Overview

    4.1 Organization

    4.2 Master Schedule

    4.3 Resources Summary

    4.4 Responsibilities

    4.5 Tools, Techniques, and Methodologies

5. Life Cycle Verification & Validation

    5.1 Management of V&V

    5.2 Concept Phase V&V

    5.3 Requirements Phase V&V

    5.4 Design Phase V&V

    5.5 Implementation Phase V&V

    5.6 Test Phase V&V

    5.7 Installation and Checkout Phase V&V

    5.8 Operation & Maintenance Phase V&V

6. Software Verification and Validation Reporting

    6.1 Required Reports

    6.2 Optional Reports

7. Verification & Validation Administration Policies

    7.1 Anomaly Reporting & Resolution

    7.2 Task Iteration Policy

    7.3 Deviation Policy

    7.4 Control Procedures

    7.5 Standards, Practices, and Conventions

Figure 9.6: Retrospective Documentation Plan—Part I

Documentation of CRF Management System Installed at XYZ Company

1. Compile a written inventory of all documentation associated with the CRF Management System at XYZ Company since its first installation. Document Examples:

   • Request for Proposal

   • Acceptance Testing Documents

   • System Manuals

   • System Logbooks

   • Maintenance Records

   • Upgrade Records

   • Code Modifications or Additions

   • User Manuals

   • Audit Reports

2. Use the above documents to establish a timeline of significant events in the Operation and Maintenance Phase of the life cycle of the CRF Management System at XYZ Company.

3. Based upon the above, write a history of the use of the CRF Management System at XYZ Company.

4. Write an overview report of user experience with the CRF Management System at XYZ Company today.

   • Who owns the system?

   • Who uses it?

   • How are access privileges given and monitored?

   • Describe today's configuration with diagrams and flow charts.

   • Document the following items:

      —Hardware & software versions

      —Maintenance & support relationships

      —Backup & disaster recovery capabilities

continued on next page

Figure 9.6 continued

—System security procedures

—Role of key users (e.g., CRA, Data Entry, etc.): what modules of the system do they use and why?

—Training available for new users & new version updates

—Software maintenance procedures

—Documentation listing: SOPs available, product manuals, user manuals, and so on

—Vendor contractual arrangements for software support and enhancements

—Any recent audit findings

5. Use a Signature Page to document Medical Management & QA review of historical and current overview reports.

6. Include an author('s) page with signatures and brief CV of relevant experience that qualifies them to know what they have written about the XYZ system experience.

Most CRF and AE management systems operate on a platform of required underlying products. These usually include a relational database, a query language to the database, security features of the hardware operating system and other items, such as separate data entry software and specific communications interfaces. It is important to identify required elements from such platform systems that are necessary for the validated performance of the CRF or AE management system.

A history should be written of the current operation of platform systems supporting the GCP validated system. A checklist for one way to address this need is given in Figure 9.7. The individual validation of Platform elements can become the objects of separate validation projects as needed. Within the Validation and Testing Plans for the CRF Management System, limits would be placed for the documentation and testing of only those Platform functions that directly affect the GCP operations of the CRF Management System.

Figure 9.7: Retrospective Documentation Plan—Part II

Documentation of Platform Systems Support for the CRF Management System Installed at XYZ Company

1. Identify the specific hardware and software elements required for validated operation of the CRF Management System at XYZ Company. These form the Platform System for the CRF software application.

   - Hardware configuration

   - Network configuration

   - Operating System elements used (e.g., security module)

   - Database software required

   - Other required software for specific functions, such as data entry, remote transmissions, or database queries

2. Compile a written inventory of all documentation associated with the Platform System hosting the CRF Management System at XYZ Company today.

   - Service contracts

   - Vendor hardware and software product manuals

   - System logbooks

   - Maintenance and support records

   - Upgrade and new version installation records

   - Code modifications or additions log

   - Data center policies and procedures for systems management

   - System backup & disaster recovery

   - Data archiving procedure

   - Physical and logical security policies

   - Personnel training and experience records

continued on next page

Figure 9.7 continued

3. Use the above documents to establish a timeline of significant events in the life of the Platform systems hosting the CRF Management System at XYZ Company today.

4. Write a report of the way Platform systems are used by the CRF Management System at XYZ Company today.

    • Which modules are reliant on platform performance?

    • How are privileges to the CRF system and Platform systems given and monitored?

    • Describe today's configuration.

        —Hardware & software versions

        —Data center and service relationship

        —Medical Department structure & functions using the CRF Management System

        —Role of key users (e.g., CRA, Data Entry, etc.): what parts of the system they use and for what purposes, such as relational database privileges or other access

        —Training available for new Platform systems support people

        —Software and hardware maintenance procedures

        —Disaster recovery & backup procedures

        —Documentation listing: SOPs available, product manuals, operations manuals, and so on.

        —Platform vendor contractual arrangements for support and enhancements: hardware, software, service, networks

        —Any recent audit findings

5. Use a Signature Page to document Medical Management & QA review of current report.

6. Include an author('s) page with signatures and brief CV of relevant experience that qualifies them to know what they have written about the XYZ Platform system experience.

GCP VALIDATION AND CANDA SUPPORT

The FDA has estimated that 80 percent of New Drug Application (NDA) data is generated during the clinical development process. This includes CRF and AE data as well as statistical analysis data sets. The

GCP validation of computerized systems managing safety and efficacy data provides a strong foundation for developing a validated computer assisted new drug application (CANDA).

The business pressure has been growing for companies to acquire the capability to deliver electronic submissions. In Europe the German BGA has an active DAMOS initiative for this. In 1992 the U.S. FDA published its CANDA Guidance Manual with the following comment in its Preface.

> The purpose of this guidance manual is to increase awareness concerning computerization and to encourage industry to computerize their NDA submissions so that we may achieve the goal of virtually all submissions being computerized by 1995. (7)

The timeliness of CANDA is becoming a current business agenda for many companies preparing to file for new product approvals in the next two years. For companies seeking definitions, the Manual defines a CANDA as

> Any automated system to improve the transmission, storage, retrieval, and/or analysis of information submitted to FDA as part of the drug development and marketing approval process. (8)

Chapter five of the FDA document is devoted to CANDA system security and integrity and covers these topics for control issues around data, software, telecommunications, hardware, and FDA interaction on CANDA projects. The connection to GCP data is quickly shown in the opening comments under data security and integrity.

> The data stored in the CANDA system represent the NDA itself. Many different components of the NDA could be stored as data—text from the NDA, document images, laboratory or patient records, or tables and graphs. Data also can be generated by the reviewer and stored in the CANDA during the course of the review.
>
> Security and integrity procedures for NDA documents should be well established within a pharmaceutical company and with FDA, and those procedures are fully applicable to CANDA system data. In addition, steps must be taken to assure consistency between the NDA hardcopy and CANDA data. (9)

A sample of FDA control issues for CANDA systems is shown in Figures 9.8 and 9.9. (10) The items covered easily apply to GCP validation efforts as well. They provide a brief view of common security and

Figure 9.8: Sample of CANDA Control Issues: Data & Software

Data Security & Integrity Controls

- Are appropriate security procedures to protect data in place at the sponsor company and FDA sites? (Access limits)

- Are CANDA data sets identical to those used to create the hardcopy NDA? Were the data validated after they were placed in the CANDA database?

- Are data change control procedures in place? Do they address changes to electronic and hardcopy data? How are corrections/changes to CRF data handled within the CANDA system?

- Is there a formal schedule for making backups of data? Are data backups stored in a secure area? Are data restore/recovery plans in place?

Software System Security & Integrity Controls

- Are security functions, such as password protection and controlled data access, built into the CANDA system?

- Does the system prohibit the FDA user from modifying the NDA data and/or CANDA system programs? Are appropriate antivirus software and procedures in place?

- Is an adequate testing plan in place to prove that the CANDA operates correctly before the system is installed at FDA? Were the internal testing and test results approved by the sponsor management?

- What plans are in place for user training and system support/enhancements? Does the CANDA have sufficient hardcopy and on-line user documentation and help information?

- Is technical system documentation available and kept up-to-date?

Figure 9.9: Sample of CANDA Control Issues: Telecom & Hardware

Telecommunications Security & Integrity Controls

- What procedures are in place to ensure accurate transmission of data via telecommunications? Are error-correcting capabilities included in telecommunications exchanges?

- Is a backup plan established for network failure? Have the following been considered for the telecommunications network?

  —Security features, such as encryption devices, dial-back modems, location and/or device ID dependent communications

  —Secure physical location of telecommunications devices and lines

  —Leased telephone lines

  —Public versus private networks

  —Password protection

  —Security violation monitoring and management reporting

Hardware Security & Integrity Controls

- Are adequate hardware security devices provided at the FDA site? Are security procedures established for CANDA hardware at the sponsor site?

- Is an identical system available for backup, testing, and/or disaster recovery? Is a disaster recovery plan in place?

- Is timely hardware maintenance available at the FDA site? Are procedures established to replenish supplies?

- If multiple CANDA systems are operating on the same machine, are appropriate security safeguards in place to allow access to authorized staff only?

control issues that need to be addressed in all systems validation efforts.

In order to have validated data in a validated CANDA, one must start with validated data at the source. This is why GCP validation of the CRF, AE, and statistical databases for a submission can provide an important foundation for a company's preparedness in doing a validated CANDA for that product.

CONCLUSION

The GCP area is a new one for computerized systems validation. It has the opportunity to benefit from the tools and techniques developed over the years for good software engineering practice and GMP and GLP validation work. This GCP validation area is characterized by ever-changing human intervention and interaction with reconfigurable computerized systems.

Each new study protocol results in software configuration changes for input screens, database structures, analysis algorithms, and randomization codes. Yet this dynamic environment holds strategic safety and efficacy data for the corporation. Validation efforts that improve the data flow and data integrity of GCP computerized systems have a major role to play in improving the time to market for new product approval and, thereby, to grow company profits.

REFERENCES

1. EC CPMP, Good Clinical Practice for Trials on Medicinal Products in the European Community (Brussels: Commission of the European Communities, 1991), p. 23.

2. Ibid.

3. EC CPMP, Biostatistical Methodology in Clinical Trials in Applications for Marketing Authorizations for Medicinal Products, Draft 4 Review Copy of CPMP Working Party Guideline (Brussels: Commission of the European Communities, March 1993), p. 16.

4. ANSI/IEEE, IEEE Standard Glossary of Software Engineering Terminology. Std 729-1983 (New York: The Institute of Electrical and Electronics Engineers, Inc., 1983), p. 35.

5. ANSI/IEEE, IEEE Standard for Software Test Documentation. Std 829-1983 (New York: The Institute of Electrical and Electronics Engineers, Inc., 1983), p. 10.

6. ANSI/IEEE, IEEE Standard for Software Verification and Validation Plans. Std 1012-1986 (New York: The Institute of Electrical and Electronics Engineers, Inc., (1986), p. 12.

7. U.S. FDA, CANDA Guidance Manual, U.S. Dept. of Health & Human Services (Washington, DC: U.S. Government Printing Office, 1992), Preface.

8. Ibid., p. 29.

9. Ibid., p. 31.

10. Ibid., pp. 31–34.

10
Computerized Laboratory Systems and GLP

Dr. Teri Stokes
International Consultant
Pharmaceutical Business Group
Digital Equipment Corporation
Basel, Switzerland

In the 1970s the essence of Good Laboratory Practice (GLP) included the quality, care, and maintenance of reagents, glassware, test equipment, and technicians. Manually updated wall charts showing performance within standard deviation ranges were sufficient to give a sense of confidence in the results coming forth from a laboratory's analytical testing activities.

Today the ever-present use of information technology (IT) in the laboratory has resulted in computerized instruments, automated data acquisition and analysis, and computer-printed reports. In the 1980s various regulatory bodies, such as the UK Department of Health (DOH), the U.S. Food and Drug Administration (FDA) and the Ministry of Health and Welfare (Koseisho) in Japan came to the conclusion that it was important to add the quality, care, and maintenance of computer systems to the list of Good Laboratory Practice concerns.

In 1990 the U.S. Environmental Protection Agency (EPA) decided that general GLPs applied to computers as "equipment" were not enough guidance for the complex world of laboratory computers in this decade. It then supplemented the GLPs by publishing a draft of the

EPA Good Automated Laboratory Practice (GALPs) regulations. How is laboratory management to cope with all this recent regulatory attention in a reasonable fashion? Here is one practical, eight-point approach.

POINT 1—INVENTORY ALL TYPES OF COMPUTER USE IN THE LABORATORY

A good way for a laboratory manager to start is to make an inventory of all computer use in the laboratory. This process includes listing all personal computers (PCs) and their use for instrument control, on-line or manual data entry, report writing, spreadsheet calculations, and so on. The lab may also have a Laboratory Information Management System (LIMS) that monitors and controls the operations of the lab as a whole.

Some laboratory facilities may have computerized HVAC (heating, ventilation, and air conditioning) systems to maintain environmental control. There may be handheld devices, such as bar code readers and scanners, in use. In addition, remote devices in the field may be used to gather testing data, perform analyses, and transmit data back to the central lab facility.

An asset inventory control number can be used to identify each computer device and this can be recorded along with the software used and lab activities performed with it. The large number of computers and computerized devices and the broad range of their use in today's laboratory can come as a surprise to many senior managers whose focus has traditionally been on the quality of reagents and proficiency of technician testing.

During this inventory one should also check for the documentation associated with each computerized system. Are there written instructions for how to use it? Is there a documented maintenance and repair record for it? Who is responsible for the system if there are problems with it? When was it last serviced?

This inventory will give management a better understanding of its use of IT and the need to more closely manage the computerized assets for both quality and business advantage. The prioritization of GLP validation efforts can then proceed based upon a specific understanding of existing computerized systems and their particular use in GLP-controlled analyses.

POINT 2—ASSESS GLP RELEVANCE FOR SPECIFIC HARDWARE AND SOFTWARE USED

The criteria for assessing the GLP relevance of computer systems are the impact on and management of data used to prove the safety, efficacy, and/or quality of a product to the regulatory authorities. Hardware and software systems that are used for the data acquisition, data entry, analysis, storage, and reporting of study data for regulatory submissions are the computerized systems to validate under GLP Standards.

This is true no matter where the computers are located. Systems used for remote data entry at another separate location or the laboratory use of host computer systems located in another building across a network remain a part of the GLP validation domain. The GLP focus is based upon system use to process, store, manage, and archive submission data for GLP-controlled studies or GMP product quality assessments.

It is appropriate for a laboratory to have a documented plan for the phased implementation of computer validation across multiple systems according to some logical lab priority for resource and risk management. This prioritization should be approved and signed by lab management and the Quality Assurance Unit (QAU). It is NOT appropriate for a laboratory to be WITHOUT a plan for validating its GLP computer systems.

A computer system hosting several software applications might have only one application coming under GLP. A system hosting financial software, word processing software, and a LIMS would have only the LIMS software application and the host hardware system to validate for GLP. The SOP-controlled operation and maintenance of the LIMS host computer system at a GLP quality level would also be to the performance benefit of other resident applications.

POINT 3—ESTABLISH A GENERAL LABORATORY QA POLICY FOR IT COMPLIANCE TO GLP STANDARDS

Developing a laboratory QA policy for GLP computer systems often requires a certain amount of cross training of disciplines for the parties concerned. The computer people need to learn about GLP regulations and how these impact computer operations. The lab people need to understand how computer procedures, or the lack thereof (in PCs for instance), can impact data integrity and GLP study compliance. And the QA Unit needs to learn more about the key issues to be monitored for regulatory compliance of computerized systems.

The GLP regulations do not allow for a double standard in their application to systems developed within the lab versus those software applications purchased from an outside vendor. Quality standards for software development according to documented engineering practices and life cycle control apply just as much to in-house programmers as to outside commercial vendors.

It is the responsibility of GLP labs to require their contracted software developers to meet GLP quality standards in their software engineering practices for regulated software applications. It is also the responsibility of GLP labs to audit the conformance of both internal and external contracted software suppliers to these standards. The lab's general QA policy for IT should acknowledge these responsibilities and state how (through which SOPs) the lab intends to fulfill these responsibilities.

POINT 4—AUDIT THE DEVELOPMENT OF IN–HOUSE AND VENDOR–SUPPLIED SYSTEMS

There are three types of computer systems to be considered for GLP review: computer systems developed in-house, systems purchased from an outside vendor, and existing systems already in operation. Existing (legacy) systems may have been further adapted with internal software to meet specific lab needs. Developing SOPs for these three cases need not be done from ground zero. There are some helpful regulatory precedents that can be used as a foundation.

The Koseisho in Japan has produced an Attachment to its GLP regulations that includes some specific recommendations for inspection of the development of internal and external computer software systems under GLP standards. See Figure 10.1 for some details of the Koseisho approach. (1)

Sections 2.A and 2.B provide guidance for assessing the prospective validation of both internal and vendor-supplied software systems. Section 2.B.5 includes systems where the laboratory has programmed additional software elements to adapt the vendor's application for its own needs. Section 2.C looks at the retrospective validation of existing systems.

These Koseisho checkpoints provide a strong guide for looking at how laboratory software has been designed and tested for GLP

Figure 10.1: Guide for GLP Inspection of Computerized Systems in Japan—Section 2.0

2.0 DEVELOPMENT OF COMPUTER SYSTEM

PURPOSE: To check that the computer system was developed to have an appropriate design and adequate capacity to function.

A. Software Developed In-House

1. Check that the testing facility has an approved development and programming standard, and check that these written standards were followed during the development.

2. For the system design specifications and system configuration specification documents, check that

    1) The computer system in which data are directly collected has the following functions that are requested under the GLP standard.

        a) Data items are recorded to include information as required by the GLP standard.

        b) Any change in computer entries is made so as not to obscure the original entry and so as to indicate the reason and the date of change, and the name of the individual responsible for the data entry.

        c) Operators can be identified. Only authorized personnel can access the system.

        d) Data integrity is secured.

    2) The system requirements specifications are satisfied.

    3) The hardware specifications in use agree with the configuration specification in the document.

    4) The configuration specifications and design specifications have been updated with each software and hardware change.

3. For the programming documents, check that

    1) Experience and qualifications of the persons who wrote the software are recorded.

    2) Programming documents (including source code) were written to allow an experienced programmer to understand the program.

continued on next page

Figure 10.1 continued

4. For the program testing documents, check that

    1) The test protocol, test results, and review and approval of the results are documented.

    2) Each function of the program is tested and the test results are recorded.

5. For the validation testing documents, check that

    1) The validation testing protocol, test results, and review and approval of the results are documented.

    2) All the problems encountered have been solved, and the treatment of these problems has been documented.

6. Check that the documents mentioned in the preceding paragraphs 1 to 5 are systematically arranged and retained as the validation documentation package to evaluate and approve the reliability of the computer system.

B. Vendor-Supplied Systems

1. Check that the specifications of the computer system are documented. Check that the computer system that collects data directly accommodates the following functions requested under the GLP standard.

    a) The data are recorded to include information as mentioned in the GLP standard.

    b) Any change in computer entries is made so as not to obscure the original entry and to indicate the reason for the change, the date, and the name of the individual responsible for the data entry.

    c) Operators can be identified and only authorized personnel can access the system.

    d) Data integrity is secured.

2. Check that the testing facility has obtained, from the outside vendor who has developed the software, the following information to confirm the reliability of the software.

    1) The information to confirm that the system has been developed according to the principles of the procedures as mentioned in section A above.

continued on next page

Figure 10.1 continued

> 2) Information on customer satisfaction history.
>
> 3) Document to confirm that the software was reviewed and approved in developmental phases.
>
> 3. For the validation testing document, check that
>
>   1) The validation testing protocol, test results, and review and approval of the results are documented.
>
>   2) All the problems encountered have been solved and recorded.
>
> 4. Check that the vendor-supplied software was changed according to the established change control procedures, and that the change has been documented and approved according to the procedures mentioned in section A above.
>
> 5. In a case where the testing facility developed a part of the system for the purpose of supporting the vendor-supplied software, check that the part of the system has been documented and approved according to procedures in section A above.
>
> 6. Check that the documents mentioned in the preceding paragraphs are systematically arranged and retained as the validation documentation package to evaluate and approve the reliability of the computer system.
>
> **C. Existing System**
>
> 1. Check that the testing facility has accomplished retrospective evaluation by reviewing the historical documentation of the system.
>
> 2. Check the testing protocols, results, records of review and approval of additional testings that were conducted to supplement paragraph C.1 to confirm the reliability of the system.
>
> 3. Check that the documents mentioned in the preceding paragraphs are systematically arranged and retained as the retrospective validation documentation package to evaluate and approve the reliability of the computer system.

compliance. Other sections of the same document discuss operation and maintenance of hardware and software, computer inspections by the QA Unit, and the suitability of computer room facilities.

For most regulated industries GLP computer validation is not a small effort. The scope and detail of testing plans and SOPs for specific labs will depend on the size and extent of computer use. This is why the first step should be an inventory of all computer use in a specific lab facility.

The commonsense factor here is that a laboratory must make a serious, documented attempt to address the assurance of GLP compliance for its computerized systems that handle data for later submission to regulatory authorities. The quality of such systems should be assessed before they are put into production use. Their continued operation should be monitored by the QA Unit to assess the ongoing quality of their performance.

POINT 5—CREATE A COLLABORATIVE PHILOSOPHY FOR QA COMPUTER AUDITS

The details of one U.S. company approach to the QA of computers can be read in an article titled "Quality assurance auditing of computer systems," written by Norbert R. Kuzel for the February 1987 issue of *Pharmaceutical Technology*. This article stresses the following philosophy for internal QA audits.

Audits are best conducted in a spirit of cooperation with the audited area, which should be encouraged to work with the audit team to try to solve mutual problems. Computerized systems are very complex, and it is easy for the audit team to overlook potential problems, especially if the audited area is making an effort to hide them. In a cooperative audit, potential problems are brought to the attention of the audit team for evaluation. An internal audit should not be a police action performed in a spirit of confrontation. (2)

The QA function can actually become a facilitator for improved productivity and better return on investment for computerized systems in the laboratory. To accomplish this, the QA activity should not consider GLP compliance as just more paperwork, but should see it as an opportunity to conduct information handling in a more effective and efficient manner for improved turnaround of testing results. GLP validation efforts should have the goal of improving the lab's business return through better control and quality of lab data that develops a more satisfied internal and external customer base for the lab's services.

The quality of computerized systems begins and ends with people. All the SOPs in the world will not solve quality issues unless the people responsible for designing, maintaining, using, auditing, and paying for the systems are positively motivated to activate the intent for quality that lies within SOPs, Validation Plans, and Audit Reports. It is important to capture the imaginations of lab scientists, technicians, and managers with the idea of GLP for computers as a collaborative mechanism for improved lab business success.

Part of the quality assurance audit procedure outlined in the Kuzel article focused on the human factors surrounding the system. This included identifying the lab community's perceptions and problems related to the system such as the following: (3)

1. User acceptance

2. Management satisfaction

3. Adequacy of up-time and response time

4. Recurrent problems and how they are handled

5. Adequacy of technical computer support

6. Adequacy of user training

7. Availability of current user manuals

8. Need for enhancements

9. Users' suggestions for improvement

This author would add a number 10 to the list: identify current system functions or services that are thought to be very useful, time/money saving, or important to quality service for lab clients. Building upon success is as important to quality improvement as correcting problems. It "feels good" to people to acknowledge the good points and this generates the enthusiasm needed to more positively handle problems.

QA units have a history of studying the people systems and paper systems of laboratories for their compliance to GLP. As they continue on with the newer elements of studying computerized data systems, they should look for ways of improving and optimizing the interaction of people, paper, and computer information flows within the lab for more efficient operations under GLP.

POINT 6—MONITOR ONGOING OPERATION AND MAINTENANCE OF REGULATED SYSTEMS

In the laboratory environment there are at least three levels of computerized systems to be considered for ongoing monitoring:

1. The database host/server systems that have LIMS types of applications for storing, analyzing, archiving, and reporting lab results

2. Automated data acquisition systems connected to analytical instruments with on-line or manual input to the database systems

3. PCs and handheld devices for the manual entry of analytical data over a communications link to the database systems

It is important that lab management establish and implement a validation policy for each level of system. These policies should state the lab's priority for GLP compliance and the rationale for deciding in which order specific systems are to be validated within each of the three levels.

After the first major validation effort for each system, there should be a plan in place to continue documented, periodic testing, and review of system operations and maintenance. When major hardware components are replaced or new versions of software are introduced, there should be a more extensive program of validation activities implemented.

Some regulated environments have too many legacy computer systems in use to validate them all immediately. In such a situation, the QA team should develop some risk assessment criteria for deciding how critical a specific system's failure would be to consumer safety, product quality, or environmental hazard. Common sense dictates that failed systems most likely to affect consumer safety are the ones to be first on the list for systems validation efforts.

The GALP document advocates the appointment of a Responsible Person for GLP systems to manage this process of ongoing systems operation, maintenance, and regulatory compliance. See Figure 10.2 for the documented GALP views on this matter. (4)

The basic message of the GALP and other GLP documents is that the computerized element of the GLP environment requires the same care and attention as other calibrated equipment would receive. Paul Lepore of the FDA elaborates on just this theme in his 1992 article, "FDA's good laboratory practice regulations and computerized data acquisition systems."

In his journal article Lepore states that

Computerized systems including hardware, software, firmware, and associated data collection and storage devices are considered to be equipment involved in a nonclinical laboratory study . . . computerized systems are subject to the equipment provisions of the good laboratory practice regulations whenever the systems are used to conduct or support a nonclinical laboratory study. (5)

Figure 10.2: EPA GALP View of Responsible Person for Lab Computers—Section 7.3

The laboratory shall designate a computer scientist or other professional of appropriate education, training, and experience or combination thereof as the individual primarily responsible for the automated data collection system(s) (the Responsible Person). This individual shall ensure that

1. There are sufficient personnel with adequate training and experience to supervise or conduct, design, and operate the automated data collection system(s). (Personnel)

2. The continuing competence of staff who design or use the automated data collection system is maintained by documentation of their training, review of work performance, and verification of required skills. (Training)

3. A security risk assessment has been made, points of vulnerability of the system have been determined, and all necessary security measures to resolve the vulnerability have been implemented. (Security)

4. The automated data collection system(s) have written operating procedures and appropriate software documentation that are complete, current, and available to staff. (SOPs)

5. All significant changes to operating procedures and/or software are approved by review and signature. (SOP Review)

6. There are adequate acceptance procedures for software and software changes. (Change Control)

7. There are procedures to assure that data are accurately recorded in the automated data collection system. (Data Recording)

8. Problems with the automated collection system that could affect data quality are documented when they occur, are subject to corrective action, and the action is documented. (Problem Reporting)

9. All applicable good laboratory practices are followed. (GALP/GLP Compliance)

Good laboratory practice regulations were first proposed by the U.S. FDA in 1976 with the objective of assuring the quality and integrity of the safety data submitted to support the approval of regulated products. Such regulated products include human and animal drugs, human biological products and medical devices, feed and food additives, and electronic products that emit radiation.

Lepore states that when the FDA looks to assess data quality, it examines five key characteristics. It expects data to be

1. *Accurate:* assuring that others can replicate the results as necessary

2. *Immediate:* recorded as soon as possible after an event is observed

3. *Legible:* written records cannot be obscure or made unreadable with crossouts and the use of opaque white-out

4. *Durable:* recorded data should be retrievable over time

5. *Attributable:* dated initials should identify the individual who collected the data (6)

When the FDA looks to assess the integrity of data, it expects the following three criteria to be met.

1. *Consistency:* Measured parameters should be within expected limits and recorded values should follow study trends.

2. *Fidelity:* Numbers and result notations should be the same wherever they are shown in study records and should keep their true value when represented as parts of means or averages.

3. *Honesty:* There is no place for fraud or misrepresentation of data in any form. (7)

The FDA expects at least the same level of quality and integrity for data collected by electronic means as for data collected manually. In practice, labs often expect more accuracy from computers that do not get bored and tired while doing repetitive data capture. This proves to be a realistic expectation when systems are properly maintained and operated according to appropriate procedures (See chapters 6 & 7).

POINT 7—PREPARE A STANDARD PROCEDURE FOR AUDITS AND INSPECTIONS

The term *audit* is usually used for company-initiated quality review activities and the term *inspection* refers to quality review by outside agencies, such as regulatory authorities or licensing groups. In either case, a company using computers in regulated environments should be prepared to facilitate a quality review "visit" of the computer systems in regulated areas.

This means preparing an SOP for how to host a quality review "visit" for regulated systems. The SOP should include the following:

- Who is notified when an auditor/inspector arrives?

- Who should meet with this reviewing individual?

- Who should accompany this person during the review?

- What systems-related documents should be easily available for review and where are they kept?

- Who authorizes the release of copies of materials to the reviewer and how is this documented?

- What company security measures are in force during the visit and what facilities are to be made available to the reviewer (e.g., designated office or conference room)?

- Who documents the content of reviewer comments during the visit and keeps copies of items copied for the reviewer?

- Who is authorized to answer technical questions about the systems, regulatory questions about GLP compliance procedures, and policy questions about company management practices in quality assurance?

- What are the corporate guidelines for the reasonability limits to reviewer questions in order to adhere to company policies on security of information?

- Where are the documents and reports relating to this visit to be kept?

In 1989 the UK Department of Health in London published its document, Good Laboratory Practice United Kingdom Compliance Program: The Application of GLP Principles to Computer Systems. This document outlines the way in which the Inspector will approach the examination of computer systems in laboratories conducting human health and environmental safety studies. (8)

It also recommends the *Red Apple Document* for detailed application of GLP principles to computer systems. (9)

The UK document explains that the Inspector will be looking for assurance that the computer systems can properly perform their assigned functions and activities. It states that this will include the following:

- Identification and functional definition of the system(s)

- Examination of control procedures

- Evaluation of effectiveness of specific functions

See Figure 10.3 for the UK GLP Compliance view of system and function inspection. (10) In addition, computer security procedures, archive management, quality assurance monitoring, and staff training will be assessed by the Inspector.

This listing of specific activities possible with UK GLP inspections shows the breadth of possible interaction required during an inspection visit. It also underscores the need for a company to think ahead and develop an SOP as previously discussed to properly manage and facilitate this process of quality review by outside agencies.

POINT 8—DOCUMENT ALL COMPLIANCE ACTIVITIES

The final recommendation for this chapter is for a company to document all activities performed for GLP compliance. Chapter 7 of this book recommends using forms to help staff remember to complete SOPs. It is also useful to see what reports the computers themselves can generate to document the monitoring of system performance.

A logical approach to managing system compliance documents is also needed. This "library" function is mentioned in Figure 10.1 as the final item on the Japanese GLP computer checklist for each type of system.

> Check that the documents mentioned . . . are systematically arranged and retained as the validation documentation package to evaluate and approve the reliability of the computer system.

Figure 10.3: UK GLP Compliance View of Inspecting Computer Systems and Functions

Identification & Functional Definition of Systems

The Inspector will normally

- Identify any parts of GLP compliant studies using a computer.

- Require definition of the hardware in use including both that used for processing and for data input and output.

- Identify the specific computer systems and subsystems in use.

- Establish the application and operating systems software, programming languages, and any other software utilities employed.

- Gather information on how the data processing function is organized, including management of operations, data capture, users, and related Quality Assurance (QA) monitoring activities.

Specific Functions

The Inspector may require details of specific functions carried out by computer (e.g., acquisition of data from an animal unit . . . or in the processing of data). This information may be obtained by

- Examination of documentation

- Examination of the methods of testing functions

- Discussion with data processing staff or users

- Requesting demonstration of specific operations

All other countries operate with the same philosophy. If an activity in a regulated environment is not documented, then it did not happen. Be sure to get full credit for your company's many efforts toward assuring the quality and integrity of its computer-resident data in regulated environments—DOCUMENT THEM!!

SUMMARY

The importance of data quality and integrity in computerized systems operating in GLP environments is recognized by regulatory authorities around the world. GLP computer inspections have been discussed in this chapter with reference to documents and directives from Europe, the United States, and Japan. All of these sources require a well-documented approach to the design, operation, and control of operations and maintenance of GLP-regulated computerized systems.

An eight-point approach to addressing these GLP validation needs has been suggested.

1. Inventory all types of computers used in the laboratory

2. Assess GLP relevance for specific hardware and software used

3. Establish a lab QA policy for computer compliance to GLP

4. Audit the development of in-house and vendor supplied systems

5. Create a collaborative philosophy for QA computer audits

6. Monitor ongoing operation and maintenance of regulated systems

7. Prepare an SOP for audits and inspections

8. Document all compliance activities

REFERENCES

1. Koseisho, "Good Laboratory Practice Attachment: GLP Inspection of Computer System," *Drug Registration Requirements in Japan*, 4th Edition (Tokyo: Yakuji Nippo, Ltd., 1991), pp. 157–159.

2. N. R. Kuzel, "Quality Assurance Auditing of Computer Systems," *Pharmaceutical Technology*, February 1987, p. 42.

3. Ibid., p. 39.

4. U.S. EPA, *Good Automated Laboratory Practices:* Recommendations for Ensuring Data Integrity in Automated Laboratory Operations with Implementation Guidance (Research

Triangle Park, NC: U.S. Environmental Protection Agency, 1990), pp. 62–76.

5. Paul D. Lepore, "FDA's good laboratory practice regulations and computerized data acquisition systems," *Chemometrics and Intelligent Laboratory Systems: Laboratory Information Management*, 1992, Vol. 17, p. 285.

6. Ibid., p. 284.

7. Ibid.

8. UK Department of Health, *Good Laboratory Practice United Kingdom Compliance Program: The Application of GLP Principles to Computer Systems* (London: Department of Health, 1989), p. 1.

9. DIA, *Computerized Data Systems for Nonclinical Safety Assessment* (Maple Glen, PA: Drug Information Association, 1988).

10. UK Dept. Health, pp. 2–3.

11

Computerized Systems Validation: Preparation for an FDA Bioprocess Inspection

Ronald C. Branning
Director, Quality Systems
Genetics, Institute, Inc.
Andover, MA, USA

The purpose of this chapter is to acquaint you with the history of regulatory requirements for computer system use and validation responsibilities for pharmaceutical manufacturers. The emphasis of this chapter will be the application of validation principles to computer controlled processes. This chapter is intended to be a step-by-step tutorial for the validation of your computerized system and preparation of the documentation for a regulatory inspection. It is a guideline for those using computerized systems in a regulated environment.

This chapter will give you a summary of the U.S. Food and Drug Administration (FDA) documentation requirements, briefly explain the basis for the regulatory position, describe the scope of validation including an outline of the considerations for software development standards, and present a model procedure and protocol for computerized system validation.

The essential message is that when the decision is made to computerize a system, the necessary expertise must be involved to ensure that the complete system is properly designed, specified, ordered, qualified, tested, operated, controlled, and monitored to keep it in a validated state. FDA requirements and industry experiences related in industry conferences, seminars, and literature articles are all detailed in the reference list at the end of this chapter. These sources should be consulted during the development of your own plan for computerized systems validation.

The reason for FDA's requirement for computerized system validation is that computer monitoring and control of critical parameters must be shown to be at least as reliable as human control. Validation has been defined as "establishing documented evidence that a process does what it purports to do." (1) What that means as a practical matter is "identifying, understanding, and controlling variability" (2) of raw materials, of the production process, in test methodology, and of product stability. Every parameter monitored and controlled by the computer must be shown to be done so with at least the same degree of assurance as shown by human operators. This means that computer control of a pharmaceutical production process, taking many parameter readings and adjusting the process according to predetermined logic, will have to be carefully and extensively tested.

Computerized system validation is the latest chapter in the history of FDA requirements for validation

Sterilization	1977–1979
Aseptic Processing	1979–1987
Water Treatment Processing	1981–1985
Nonaseptic Processing	1983–1987
Computer Related Systems	1983–?

that have been superbly documented by Ken Chapman. (3)

The use of computers to monitor and control production processes is incorporated in the *Code of Federal Regulations*, Food and Drugs 21, Part 211, Current Good Manufacturing Practice for Finished Pharmaceuticals (GMPs) Subpart D, Equipment, Section 211.68 "Automatic, mechanical, and electronic equipment." The FDA *Compliance Policy Guides* have supplemented the GMPs for specific reference to documentation, records, source code, testing and vendor responsibility. (4) Therefore, the requirement for validation of computerized systems is the law. Furthermore, several FDA spokesmen, including Commissioner Kessler, have stated in industry forums in 1991 that New Drug Applications will be approved only if the process is validated.

The enforcement of the regulations is carried out by a number of trained FDA specialists who examine a firm's computerized systems usually in conjunction with routine facility inspections. These are the questions you can expect the FDA inspector to ask concerning your computerized systems:

- Do you have an SOP for computerized system validation?

- Is there a list of all computers used in this facility?

- Does each computer have a defined set of functions?

- Have knowledgeable technicians and management reviewed the list of computers and functions to determine which computerized systems require validation?

- For those computerized systems that you have determined require validation, is there a validation schedule?

- Are there validation protocols for those computerized systems?

- Do you have a validation summary report for each completed protocol?

- Has QA audited the validation documentation?

- Is there a process monitoring and change control system in place to maintain the computerized system in a validated state?

- Has management approved the computerized system as validated and acceptable for use?

These questions are the initial outline of the requirements for computerized systems validation. Let us take them in sequence to prepare a step-by-step approach. The two key documents are an SOP for computerized system validation and a validation protocol.

SOP FOR COMPUTERIZED SYSTEM VALIDATION

The SOP should contain these elements:

Objective: Computerized system validation.

Scope: Appropriate facility or business entity description.

Definitions: Computer, computerized system, validation, and other key words defined for the people who will have to use this SOP.

Responsibility: Each department or position responsibility should be delineated, especially for

Management Information Systems (MIS)
R&D
Production
QC Laboratories
Quality Assurance
Management

Procedure:

1. Identification of all computers and computerized systems used by the firm defined by the **SCOPE** of this SOP.

2. Definition of the function of all computers and computerized systems on the list.

3. Criteria for validation (examples):

    a. Critical system monitoring/control.

    b. Raw data retrieval, storage or manipulation.

    c. Critical document control (Batch records, test methods, SOPs).

    d. Computerized (paperless) inventory control.

4. Establishment of a Computerized Systems Validation Committee (CSVC) to decide which computers and computerized systems require validation. This committee should include MIS, R&D, Materials, Production, QA, and QC.

5. CSVC priorities and schedule for validation.

6. Protocol requirements.

COMPUTERIZED SYSTEM VALIDATION PROTOCOL

The validation protocol should follow the SOP with the details and responsibilities stated clearly. The requirements for completing this protocol are the same for a currently operating installed system as for one that is being proposed or designed. The difference is that existing data would be gathered from the files to be used for installed systems; incomplete information would have to be updated. The protocol should contain at least these sections:

Responsibilities: Specific individuals should be designated by name and title as being responsible for significant parts of the validation.

Basis of Design: The computer and computerized system functions should be completely described.

Specifications: Specifications for the computer, including software, and the equipment and/or instrumentation it will be connected to should be detailed.

Installation Qualification: The installation of the computer, including software, and the equipment and/or instruments should be verified against the specifications.

Training: Training manuals, including manufacturer/supplier instructions, should be used to develop operational instructions (SOPs) and training classes for operators and technicians.

Operational Qualification: The installed computer, including software, and the various pieces of equipment and/or instrumentation should be calibrated or otherwise set up and shown to operate independently within their expected parameters.

Performance Qualification: The computerized system (comprising the computer, including software, the equipment and/or instrumentation) functions correctly as a unit through a series of preliminary trials.

Testing: System test plans should be developed prospectively for the validation trials. QC test methods for materials and products should be validated prior to the validation trials.

Validation: The computerized system should be put through a preplanned series of tests to demonstrate that the system not only functions as it did in the preliminary trials, but performs acceptably all the critical functions defined in the **Basis of Design.** Product produced should be shown to meet all its quality requirements. Tests performed with computerized laboratory equipment should be shown to be comparable to manual testing. Data storage and manipulation should be shown to be equivalent to manual recording and calculation.

Results Analysis: A technically competent member of the validation team should review the data and write a summary report of the validation test results.

Change Control: Specific process monitoring and change control provisions should be made for this system. A periodic review, at least annually, should be set up to ensure that it is maintained in a validated state.

QA Audit: QA should audit the documentation for compliance to the SOP and review the data to ensure that the system test plans meet the requirements of the **Basis of Design** and that the results support the conclusions. The computer/computerized system should then be added to the internal audit schedule.

Management Approval: Management should formally sign-off the validation report, officially designating the system as validated and acceptable for use.

DEFINITIONS

Computers have become necessary components of pharmaceutical systems that control operations in R&D, Production, QA/QC, and Materials Management. The fact that they handle so much critical data and decision support information makes the validation of computerized systems imperative.

A computerized system is made up of several components. For our purposes there are several definitions that are necessary in order to understand the principles of computerized systems validation:

- **Computer Hardware (HW)** means the mainframe, mini, or portable computer.

- **Software (SW)** is categorized as either operating software or applications software. *Operating software* sets up the computer hardware to run and accept the instructions of applications software. *Applications software* includes programs written for specific functions, such as data gathering (bioreactor sensors), process control (pumps on/off) data analysis (statistics on QC test results), document control (batch records, SOP, Test Methods) and graphics (QC control charts).

- **Equipment** is usually the designation given to process items such as a bioreactor and the probes, sensors, pumps, and other accessory support pieces.

- **Instruments** are generally associated with in-line or QC testing (GC, HPLC).

- **Computerized system,** therefore, means the total configuration: computer hardware, software, and the associated equipment and/or instrumentation.

REGULATORY ENVIRONMENT

The FDA recognized prior to 1983 that computers were being extensively used in the critical data gathering and control functions within the industry. In order to determine how to effectively begin the process of regulating them, the FDA recruited specialists in computers and computerized systems and developed the "Blue Book." (5) They also selected a number of investigators from the various districts to attend special classes to learn about computers and their use in the pharmaceutical industry. These specialists have been loaned out to the local districts for specific assignments. These specialists found significant deficiencies in the pharmaceutical industry's control of computerized systems.

Wyeth's nonclinical lab in Malvern, Pennsylvania, was the first widely reported FDA computerized system inspection. It put the industry on notice that the FDA was serious about pharmaceutical computer systems validation. (6)

The Pharmaceutical Manufacturers Association (PMA) organized the first Computer Systems Validation Seminar in Washington in January 1984. At that meeting the formation of the PMA Computer Systems Validation Committee was announced. The committee proceeded to publish a watershed article in *Pharmaceutical Technology,* "Validation Concepts for Computer Systems Used in the Manufacture of Drug Products" (7), which changed and clarified the pharmaceutical manufacturer's view of computerized systems for their production applications.

A second landmark inspection occurred in 1985 at Boehringer Ingelheim's production facility in Ridgefield, Connecticut; this inspection resulted in a number of FD-483 citations. (8) The details of those criticisms and the subsequent successful computerized dispensing system inspection have been shared with the pharmaceutical, medical device, chemical, and other industry groups through a series of lectures and seminars. The information was shared in order to provide a factual base for the discussion of the requirements for compliance to FDA CGMP and thus keep other firms from having to "reinvent the wheel" for their computerized systems validation.

There have been a number of meetings and seminars during the past seven years sponsored by the PMA, *Pharmaceutical Technology* (*Pharm. Tech.*), the International Society for Pharmaceutical Engineering

(ISPE), the Parenteral Drug Association (PDA), the American Society for Quality Control (ASQC), the American Chemical Society (ACS), and others to help formulate practical approaches to computerized systems validation. The proceedings of these conferences may be obtained directly from the sponsoring organization. There are also a number of introductory and advanced computerized system validation topics currently being offered by these same organizations.

The FDA has incorporated computerized system validation as part of their routine inspection checklist. So you can expect to be asked a number of questions about the status of your computerized systems during your next biannual inspection.

INITIAL CONSIDERATION FOR SYSTEM COMPUTERIZATION

The reliance on computers has risen dramatically in the past 10 years because most of us equate the use of computers with reliability and speed. The fact is, however, that computers only do what they are designed (hardware) to do and told (programmed software) to do. If you are not sure exactly what you want a specific computerized system to do, then it will not be appropriately designed and programmed; the system will not work the way you imagined unless you can completely visualize and carefully specify the system. The best way to approach such a project is to determine what you think you want, then get someone with expertise in computer systems to help you clarify your thoughts and assist you in writing specifications for your system.

A typical example of the problems encountered in attempts to computerize critical systems is a pharmaceutical firm that spent more than $250,000 for hardware and software during a 2-year project. The computer system eventually had to be replaced because the hardware was not properly specified and the software had so many faults it never worked. This incident also illustrates why the FDA is so interested in the computer systems that control the production and testing of pharmaceuticals.

To avoid this type of problem, some preliminary steps should be taken to clarify and justify computer control of your system:

Scope

The scope of the computerized system must be defined in order to determine its technical feasibility and financial justification. The first question you must ask is, "What are we trying to do?" The answer must be written down primarily to clarify the project in the mind of the project sponsor. The scope should include both existing and future requirements for the budget. All of the project team members and selected management should review and approve the project scope.

Graphical Presentation

Once the written scope is completed, a preliminary picture of the project should be developed, such as a diagram labeled with the process equipment and connections to the computer hardware. This may sound like a unnecessary step, but I have been involved in many situations where team members had completely opposite ideas of how a system was to function simply because they had never drawn a picture of it. Ultimately, a well-labeled picture of the computerized system including the computer, software details, and the associated equipment and/or instrumentation will be worth more than a thousand words when describing it to the FDA.

Input/Output

The input/output requirements will help determine the specifications for operating and applications software. Input means the way data will go into the computer database. Output means the way data will be manipulated and printed out in reports. Simulated output should be developed by the project sponsor to help the other team members, especially the programmers, see what success will look like.

Flow Chart/Critical Point Analysis

The written scope and graphical presentation should be further refined in a sequence flow chart with critical monitoring and control points identified. These key points are the basis of the decisions concerning what and how much computerization will be needed.

Cost Analysis

Cost-effectiveness of computerization should be based on the productivity and product quality improvement anticipated with computer control versus human monitoring and control. The comparison should also be made between the quantity and quality of the data collected by computers versus that which can be documented by people. There is no argument, however, that the computer can collect and analyze vast amounts of data and present it in far more meaningful forms much faster than humans. The development of "expert systems" software also gives computers an edge in the diagnosis and correction of process problems.

If the immediate cost of computerization and eventual benefits do not balance, then serious consideration should be given to manual control or limited automatic monitoring with manual control. However, there are some processes that are too critical and/or complicated to be completely manually controlled regardless of the cost analysis.

Supplier Control Systems

There are a number of firms that offer "turn-key" specification, installation, and validation services for computerized control systems for their equipment, instruments, processes, and environmental support systems. These services should be critically reviewed in light of the information provided in this chapter.

SPECIFYING COMPUTER SYSTEMS

Once the decision has been made to purchase a computerized system or computerize an existing one, then the appropriate people must get together to plan the project:

- Project sponsor—the head of the team

- R&D, Production, or QC—a representative from the department who will use the system

- MIS—who will provide the computer technical expertise

- QA—for regulatory compliance auditing

These people will have to spend a significant amount of time developing detailed specifications. This will be time well spent since studies conducted by DEC and IBM indicate savings of 25–50 percent of total project costs by following a structured approach to development with emphasis on initial planning. (9)

PMA LIFE CYCLE APPROACH

The PMA Computer Systems Validation Committee developed a life cycle approach as part of their 1986 position paper. (Figure 11.1) The following steps are compatible with this structured approach to

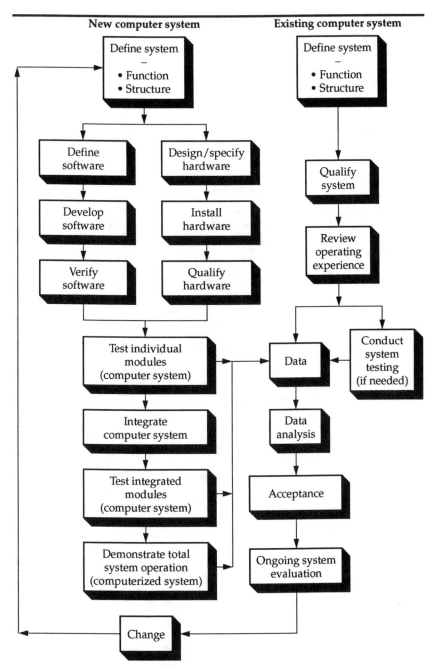

Figure 11.1. Validation life cycle approach. (Source: Pharmaceutical Manufacturers Association Computer Validation Committee, Validation Concepts for Computer Systems Used in the Manufacture of Drug Products. *Pharm. Tech.***, September 1986.)**

development, continuing evaluation, monitoring, and control of pharmaceutical computerized systems.

System Definition

At this point it is necessary to split the project into two components:

1. equipment/instrumentation/process

2. computer hardware/software

The preceding preliminary design information should all be updated and used for the development of final requirements that can be turned into specifications. The project needs to be divided because the expertise is different for each part. Both still need to be closely coordinated since the process and/or instrumentation will be monitored and controlled by the computer system; validation will encompass the complete computerized system.

Purchase Specifications

The detailed design requirements should be converted into purchase specifications for the equipment, instruments, hardware, and software. Internal service requests, purchase orders, and contracts should have the appropriate sections of the detailed design specifications attached as further clarification of the requirements.

Equipment/Instrumentation/Process

The requirements for equipment, instrumentation and process validation are beyond the scope of this chapter however the principles are the same as those for computerized systems.

Computer Hardware/Software

Hardware Selection

Hardware selection is usually simpler than software selection if only in relative terms. Most computer (MIS) departments have a standard hardware platform for specific applications; if not, there are usually compatibility constraints. The primary considerations for the selection are compatibility, capacity both in RAM and disk storage, user requirements and sophistication, speed, cost, and convenience. The better the definition of user requirements related to the tasks, the easier the selection of the hardware.

Software Development Standards

Off-the-shelf software can be purchased for a number of functions. Many of these so called "configurable" programs allow you to insert your requirements for parameter monitoring and control (i.e., temperature monitored within limits; out of range conditions alarm). The number of parameters that can be measured and the report formats are usually fixed by the program, but the specific functions and ranges are selected by the user. Custom software must be developed by in-house or contract programmers for applications that are beyond the capability of "configurable" software.

Since the FDA considers source code to be part of master production and control records and the process control via software functions will have to be validated, it is imperative that a set of standards be used in the development of applications software. Software development standards must be the same for both configurable and custom applications software. Software development is the heart of computerized process validation because you have to build quality into the software, it cannot be tested into the final program.

Software Development Standards Outline

This is a suggested ten-step approach to the development of good software documentation elements that will support software verification as part of an overall process validation protocol:

1. **Project Definition:** The project sponsor should review the detailed design with those responsible for programming and supervising the development of the application program.

2. **Requirements Definition:** The requirements should be defined from the preceding **Scope** and **Graphical Presentation** information by both the project sponsor and the programmers.

3. **Conceptual Design:** The conceptual design should be prepared by the programmers and reviewed and approved by their supervisors and the project sponsor. This design should include required outputs, data input, the processing required to create the output, and a conceptual system flow chart.

4. **Detailed System Design:** Once the conceptual design has been approved, a detailed design should be prepared by

the programmers and their supervisor for the review and approval by the project sponsor. This design should include proposals for output format, flow charts, decision tables, program security, data editing and decision rules, and audit trails.

After the project sponsor has approved the detailed design, a software verification plan for the validation protocol should be prepared by the programmers for their supervisor's approval. This plan should include the requirements for programming language, program flow chart, English language explanation of the various module's functions, a test plan, test/modification/retest documentation requirements, and supervisory review and approval at key stages of programming.

5. **Hardware Installation Certification:** Where possible, the hardware platform that will be used in the computerized process validation should be used to develop the applications software. The hardware should be installed, diagnostically tested, and certified by the hardware supplier.

6. **Programming Specifications:** The modules and the function and specifications for each module should be developed at this stage.

7. **Programming:** Each module should be programmed, compiled, and corrected as necessary.

8. **Programming Test/Software Verification:** The modules should be tested and documented according to the validation protocol test plan. Program corrections and modifications should be appropriately tested and documented. The program's source code and the test data should be reviewed and approved by the programmer's supervisor.

9. **System Test:** The program should be tested according to the validation protocol with test data. The simulated inputs and actual outputs should be checked against expected outputs. Modifications should be appropriately tested and documented. The documentation package should be reviewed and approved by the programmer's supervisor and the project sponsor.

10. **Implementation:** The approved applications program should be installed in the process control computer and tested according to the validation protocol. The results of the testing should be audited according to the validation protocol and approved by Quality Assurance. Production management should also indicate approval prior to the initiation of production with a new computerized process monitoring/control system.

Verified applications software is validatable when developed according to the above guidelines, when used in conjunction with certified computer hardware and a performance qualified process. The validation protocol for the process should specify the requirements for functionally testing the operation of the process and the quality of the product that is produced. Consistent product quality is the ultimate test for computerized process validation.

Installation Qualification

The process equipment, instrumentation, computer hardware, and software that was ordered according to detailed design requirements needs to be double-checked to ensure that the items delivered match those specified. Installation qualification is nothing more than checking to be sure that what you ordered is what you received. The actual installation can be performed by the supplier and/or your contractor. The documentation of installation qualification constitutes part of the validation protocol.

Procedures and Training

Procedures (SOPs) should be developed or modified for all aspects of process operations and control. Operators and technicians should receive their initial training in the SOPs so that they can develop some process control expertise. By participating in the operational qualification and performance qualification trials, they will receive valuable on-the-job training.

Operational Qualification

Operational qualification simply means that after the process equipment, instrumentation, and computer hardware and software is installed, that it works as expected. Process equipment qualification usually relates to speed, temperature, time, and volume parameters.

Instrument qualification centers around calibration, precision, accuracy, and reproducibility. There are specific diagnostic programs supplied by the vendor for computer hardware and operating system software to ensure proper computer system functions. The applications software verification has been described previously in detail.

Performance Qualification

Performance qualification is the demonstration that the computerized process in place performs the functions originally specified in the design. While operational qualification is the exercise of the component parts of the process system by themselves, performance qualification is the demonstration that each component in the system performs its functions in sync with all the other components. Performance qualification should not be confused with validation testing. Performance qualification is the functional assurance that the system works; validation is the repetitive testing of those functions, including making sure that the system operates in a state of control within predetermined parameters.

Validation

The computerized system should be put through a preplanned series of tests documented in the validation protocol to demonstrate that the system not only functions as it did during the performance qualification trials but performs all the functions defined in the detailed design. For example,

50 L Bioreactor Temperature Control

Design Temperature Range	0°–100°
Operating Temperature Range	25°–40°

Installation qualification should have determined that the system installed was the one specified. Operational qualification should have verified that the temperature control on the bioreactor operated over the range of 0°–100°. Performance qualification should have ensured that the computer monitoring and control system, including the sensors and other support systems, worked together over the designed temperature range. Validation confirms the reproducibility of the system—that it can be controlled in the operating range during production. Product produced during validation trials should be shown to meet all of its quality requirements.

Change Control

The validated computerized process must be appropriately maintained and repaired. Periodic, usually annual, reviews of the process are required to ensure that it is kept in a validated state. Procedures should be in place for all activities related to maintenance and repair; significant changes to the process equipment, instrumentation, or computerized control should be formally authorized through a change control procedure.

Summary

Computerized systems validation begins with the requirements for pharmaceutical processing. The validation trials are simply test plans that demonstrate that the process variables defined in the detailed design are under control and that the process consistently produces acceptable product.

COMPUTER CONTROL OF BIOREACTOR PROCESSING

Validation is a journey, not a destination. A process cannot be developed, run "successfully" 3–5 times, and be declared to be validated—even if it produces a product that meets specifications. The simplistic approach of batch-to-batch product consistency is usually proposed because of ignorance of the productivity and financial benefits of validation. The primary reason for this uninformed opinion is that validation is in many cases an afterthought in the registration process for new products. If validation is attempted as an event at the end of process development, then the myth that validation requires too much time, takes too many people, and costs too much becomes a self-fulfilling prophesy. A validation template must be created for the organization so that all efforts are directed at identifying, understanding, and controlling variability. The template should include standard formats for the required validation documentation based on SOPs and protocols. (Figure 11.2)

Cell Line Validation

The validation of a bioreactor process begins during the selection of the cell line and the development of the process to produce the desired

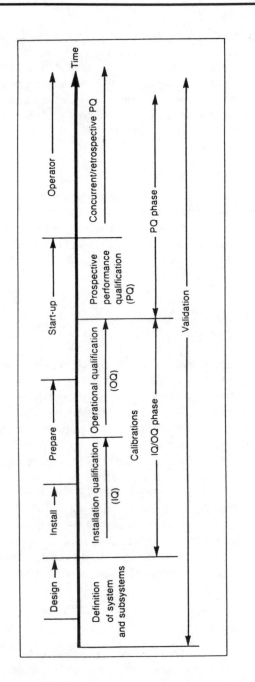

Figure 11.2. The validation time line. (Source: Chapman, K. C., A History of Validation in the United States—Part I. *Pharm. Tech.*, Oct 1991.)

protein. Cell line validation is beyond the scope of this chapter; however, suffice it to say that complete characterization and virus validation are necessary components of the complete validation picture.

Facility Certification

The facility for the production of biopharmaceuticals should be certified based on the requirements for an aseptic facility. The specifics are adequately described in the literature; however, these are some points that should be considered:

- Special attention should be given to the production room finishes for cleanability. Cleaning procedures must be validated.

- The HVAC system must be designed to provide appropriate air quality to the various areas, prevent cross-contamination, and provide isolation as required.

- Environmental monitoring and control SOPs are necessary.

- The Water for Injection (WFI) system must be validated.

- The potable water, waste disposal, and sewer systems must be validated to ensure acceptable incoming water supply and no contamination by cross-connection with the waste disposal and sewer system.

Raw Materials

Raw materials must be completely specified; the test methods for their analysis validated. A raw material supplier selection, approval, and certification process should be in place to ensure a continuing source of acceptable starting materials.

Equipment and Instrumentation

Equipment and instrumentation should be selected by an optimum equipment selection process based on the product and production requirements. A vendor qualification process similar to that for raw materials should be established to make sure that the equipment company has the knowledge and experience in the biopharmaceutical industry to meet the needs of your process.

Equipment should be designed not only for efficient operation but also for ease of cleaning, sanitization, and sterilization. Clean-in-place/sterilize in place systems (CIP/SIP) must be validated.

Process monitoring and control systems should be selected as carefully as equipment. Many equipment suppliers have control systems that are included in their proposals. A word of caution about these "complete package" systems is that the equipment suppliers have contractors for the monitoring and control computer hardware. In many cases the hardware supplier has a third-party relationship with a software programmer. Therefore, if you have problems, you could be dealing with three suppliers not one. Be sure you clearly understand the system and the relative risks before you commit to a contract.

Test Methods

Test methods, developed as part of a technology transfer package, must be capable of being utilized in a production laboratory. This means that the development and production laboratories must collaborate in the validation of raw material, in-process and finished product, and stability indicating methods.

Bioprocess Validation

Computerized control of bioprocesses is necessary because a properly programmed monitoring and control computer can make process adjustments more effectively and efficiently than manual control. As support for this position, during a presentation by an equipment manufacturer at an industry meeting, data was displayed that indicated a 10–15 percent increase in productivity using computer monitoring and control. While this is only one example, it seems reasonable. With this basic information let us look at a recent application of statistics to validation that will allow us to optimize and validate the process at the same time by using designed experiments. The details of experimental design are described in two books included in the references. (10, 11)

Given that the basic requirements for validation are in place—certified facility, validated systems, certified raw materials, qualified equipment, calibrated instrumentation, certified computer hardware, verified software, trained operators, and validated test methods—then the process is ready for product optimization and validation. As mentioned before, identifying, understanding, and controlling variability is the purpose of validation. For simplicity we will consider dissolved oxygen (DO), temperature (TEMP) and media flow rate (MFR) as the three most critical variable factors affecting both product quality and process productivity. The initial target (T), highest (H) and lowest (L) reasonable operating values for these three factors are then determined and set up in a matrix for test runs.

RUN	DO	TEMP	MFR	PRODUCTIVITY	QUALITY
1	T	T	T	100%	100%
2	L	L	L		
3	L	L	H		
4	L	H	L		
5	L	H	H		
6	H	L	L		
7	H	L	H		
8	H	H	L		
9	H	H	H		

The target values should be used for the initial run to establish a baseline for the evaluation of the remaining runs. The high and low values should be used in the succeeding runs with all other parameters being held constant. Analysis of the results will indicate the optimum process settings. These optimum settings should then be used as the new targets and new high and low reasonable operating values for additional runs, if necessary. This methodology will give you the optimum process running conditions. Once you have established the high and low operating ranges, you will have also met the requirements for validation. The process can now be run in control and with confidence. (Figure 11.3)

This methodology generally requires less than half the time of a conventional "one-factor-at-a-time" or "hit and miss" approach. The process productivity in several cases was greater than 25 percent and product quality was significantly improved. The additional fact that at the end of this project the process is validated means that this is the best methodology to use.

CONCLUSION

The FDA insists that process validation is a necessary requirement for NDA approval, but they also ask for current process validation documentation. Even though computerized systems are the best way to monitor and control complex processes, their validation can be

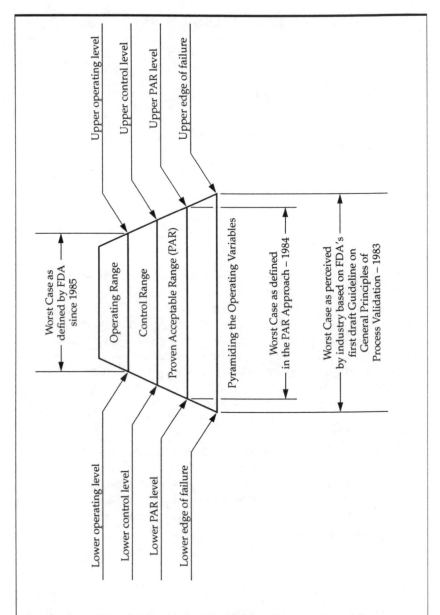

Figure 11.3. Pyramiding parameters and worst case. (Source: Chapman, K. C., A History of Validation in the United States—Part I. *Pharm. Tech.***, Oct 1991.)**

difficult. The information provided in this chapter is a starting point for the development of your validation program.

REFERENCES

1. Chapman, K. C., A History of Validation in the United States—Part I. *Pharm. Tech.*, Oct 1991.

2. Branning, R., Validation by Design—Designed Experiments for Pharmaceutical Development, Validation, Manufacturing and Quality. *Pharmaceutical Technology Conference,* 1991.

3. Chapman, 1991.

4. FDA, *Compliance Policy Guides:* 7132a.11 (1984), 7132a.12 (1985), 7132a.15 (1987).

5. FDA, Guide to Inspection of Computerized Systems Used in Manufacturing of Drug Products (*The Blue Book*), February 1983.

6. *The Gold Sheet*, January 1985.

7. Pharmaceutical Manufacturers Association Computer Validation Committee, Validation Concepts for Computer Systems Used in the Manufacture of Drug Products. *Pharm. Tech.*, September 1986.

8. *The Gold Sheet*, August 1986.

9. European Organization for Quality (EOQC), *First European Seminar on Software Quality*, April 1988.

10. Box, G. E. P., W. G. Hunter, J. Stewart Hunter, *Statistics for Experiments*. J. Wiley and Sons, Inc. 1978.

11. Haaland, P. D., *Experimental Design in Biotechnology*. Marcel Dekker, Inc. 1989.

12
Organization and Training for Validation

Ronald C. Branning
Director, Quality Systems
Genetics Institute, Inc.
Andover, MA, USA

REGULATORY REQUIREMENTS

World health authorities have developed guidelines and regulations over the past thirty years that provide the foundation for biopharmaceutical industry compliance—what is required but not necessarily how to comply. International regulations are consistent in that an appropriate level of managerial and operational competence (education, training, and experience) is expected in the manufacture of healthcare products. It is anticipated that firms will do the necessary things correctly in order to attain product approval and maintain an acceptable compliance status. This chapter addresses the methodology for identifying and setting up a Validation Master Plan and corresponding training practices to ensure computer related systems validation compliance.

VALIDATION MASTER PLAN (VMP)

The best way to approach a large, complex task, such as validation, is with a well-developed plan. Since validation approaches and details are interpreted by each firm based on its body of knowledge, degree of sophistication, and availability of resources, each company will have a different plan; however, the content, direction, and intent should be the same.

Given the increasing emphasis on validation by the health authorities, a Validation Master Plan (Figure 12.1) is necessary for compliance; it is a road map that indicates where you are, where you need to go, and the necessary steps along the way.

VMP Summary

The Validation Master Plan (VMP) is a summary of all validation activities related to a corporation or a single facility; it is an overall plan for validation. World health authority Good Manufacturing Practice regulations and industry guidelines related to validation should be used as the basis for the plan. The references and suggestions in this book are good sources. The development of your plan should be undertaken with great care and over enough time to allow the organization to assimilate it as a tool to use productively, as opposed to being another layer of bureaucracy.

The major components of the VMP for a given firm should include the following:

Facilities

The facility should be designed to meet world regulatory requirements since most companies are currently or will eventually be engaged in international markets. The recognition of this fact and the preparation for it must be formulated by a cross functional team consisting of representatives from Engineering, Maintenance, Research, Development, Manufacturing, Quality, and Regulatory Affairs. These same team members will also be essential to the development and implementation of the VMP.

Research

Research documentation of the discovery of novel compounds for therapeutic use should not only be looked at as the basis for patent protection but also as foundation validation information. Since the essence of

Figure 12.1. Validation Master Plan		
Document	**Authorship/Responsibility**	**Approval**
Corporate VMP	Corporate/Headquarters	President Corporate VPs
Facility VMP	Local Facility Staff	Local VPs Directors
Facility Certification	Functional Department Heads • Local • National • International	Responsible Head
Functional Area Validation Master Plans	Functional Departments Heads • Engineering • Maintenance • Cell Culture • Purification • Analytical Development • Production • Quality Control • Quality Assurance	Responsible Head Local VPs Local Directors
IQ/OQ/PQ Protocols	Functional Departments	Functional Heads
Monitoring/ Change Control Programs	Functional Departments	Functional Heads

validation is knowledge, understanding and control of variability everything noted during the discovery process is valuable building material for validation.

Process Development

Process development activities transform research discoveries into small-scale production and purification of the protein of interest for clinical studies. These activities continue to construct the validation record on the firm foundation established by Research.

Product Development

Product development activities prepare the biological drug substance for animal and human clinical trials. These activities are crucial to validation requirements since the health authorities require at least process and product consistency, if not validation, by the end of clinical trials and prior to product licensing.

Commercial Production

Commercial production processes are expected not only to be validated but also to be maintained in a state of control. This means that substantial effort and documentation is required to develop, implement, and maintain a change control program.

Quality

Quality systems that identify, monitor, control, and assess the development, manufacturing, and purification of proteins and production of finished products is essential to the validation effort.

Regulatory Affairs

Regulatory Affairs must be involved at each stage of the product's life to ensure that the firm and the regulators have appropriate communications.

Other departments or functions may need to be included depending on the company's particular organizational structure or functions; the necessity to develop a complete plan should determine the list of participants.

Computer Related Systems Validation—Organization

Computer related systems validation fits into the overall scheme of validation master planning as noted in Figure 12.2.

A Validation Council consisting of representatives from Engineering, Maintenance, Research, Development, Manufacturing, Quality, and Regulatory Affairs should oversee the development of Functional Area VMPs to implement the corporate/facility plan. The foundation of Research data, the building upon it by subsequent departments, and the dependence and interrelationship of each department's data on all others becomes evident as the plan is formulated. The parts have to come together like the assembled pieces of a puzzle.

Individual functional area VMPs consist of the details of each department's contribution to the validation effort. The information about the product and sources of variability becomes more detailed

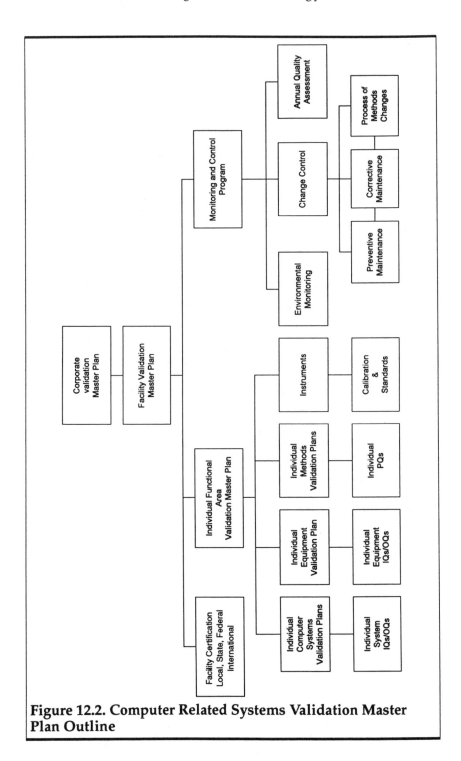

Figure 12.2. Computer Related Systems Validation Master Plan Outline

along the journey from discovery to licensure. Therefore, the significance of data and the level of documentation needs to be appropriately
described for each functional area in relation to the others. There needs
to be a "handshake" between departments as a process moves along
the path to approval. The documentation is sometimes called a
Technology Transfer Package.

The necessary validation components of concept, specification,
design, and IQ/OQ/PQ are more than adequately described in other
chapters. The take home message of this chapter is that at the end of
the day all these parts of validation must come together. They cannot
unless those responsible for validation insist that the participants are
prepared through training to carry out the company's expectations for
validation.

Computer Related Systems Validation—Training Program

Computer related systems validation is defined appropriately by the
other authors in this book. By way of review, the ten basic steps for
success in validating computer related systems are as follows:

1. Read the regulations and the references in this book.

2. Form a multidisciplinary group to address validation.

3. Establish a Policy, SOPs, and a Validation Master Plan.

4. Develop a training system and appropriate infrastructure.

5. Inventory the computer related systems.

6. Determine validation requirements and priorities.

7. Develop protocol templates/write and execute protocols.

8. Technical validation review/approval.

9. Quality Assurance validation review/approval.

10. Management validation review/approval.

This section focuses on step four—the training scheme; one approach is
outlined in Figure 12.3:

Core Training

The basic courses in regulatory requirements should be delivered to all
employees. The program should be based on local, national, and international regulations. Industry guidelines and standards are also an
excellent source of ways to approach training. The company must then
interpret its philosophy of compliance through Standard Operating
Procedures (SOPs) developed by the firm. The resulting Good

Personnel Category	Core GMP/GLP/GCP (Same for all)								Job Specific (Different for each job)								Targeted Training/Retraining for Computer Related Systems Validation					
	I	I	III	IV	V	VI	VII	VIII	A	B	C	D	E	F	G	H	Train the Trainer	Regulations/ Guidelines	Policy/ SOPs	Technical Writing	Internal/ Vendor Audit Techniques	Mgt "Hot" Topics
Management	X	X	X	X	X	X	X	X	X	X	X	X	X	X	X	X	X	X	X	X	X	X
Functional Heads	X	X	X	X	X	X	X	X	X	X	X	X	X	X	X	X	X	X	X	X	X	
Group Leaders/ Scientists	X	X	X	X	X	X	X	X	X	X	X	X	X	X	X	X	X	X	X	X	X	
Specialists/ Technicians/ Operators	X	X	X	X	X	X	X	X	X	X	X	X	X	X	X	X	X	X	X	X		

Figure 12.3. Computer Related Systems Validation Training Matrix

Manufacturing Practice courses should form the core of the compliance curriculum and should be essentially the same for all employees.

Job Function Specific

Each position requires specific training to ensure competent execution of responsibilities. This portion of the training program should not only be tailored to various functions but also to the different levels in the organization.

Each position should be defined with regard to education, training, and experience requirements. Individuals filling these positions should have their profile matched against the requirements for the job. Since there is never a perfect match, deficiencies should be defined in a written plan for bringing that individual up to the requirements of a specific job. This technique can also be used as a tool for developing training programs that reflect the organization's needs. In training jargon this is known as a needs analysis; it identifies for the trainers a profile of what the positions are, who the people are in those positions, and their training needs.

Special emphasis should be given to supervisors and managers. Train the trainer seminars are needed for supervisors since this is their essential role. Managers should be updated on the latest regulatory "hot topics" and be reminded of their continuing responsibility to support the training infrastructure.

Computer Related Systems Validation Training

Initial training for the participants in computer related systems validation is in addition to the programs mentioned above. After the completion of the first round of training, these courses can be segmented and incorporated into the core and job specific portions of the overall training scheme.

The various segments of the Targeted Training listed in Figure 12.3 (Train the Trainer, Regulations/Guidelines, Policy/SOPs, Technical Writing, Internal/Vendor Audit Techniques, Management "Hot" Topics) are examples used by one company. The curriculum should be developed specifically for the individual needs of your firm.

Management's Role in Training. The regulatory authorities hold management responsible and accountable for everything that goes on in biopharmaceutical manufacturing operations. This means that management must be trained so they understand that their responsibility is not to wait for things to happen; they must, in fact, be actively involved in making them happen. Management must fully support the entire training program not only as it relates to GMPs, but also as it promotes management and staff competence.

Regulatory Audit Training. Each employee trained according to the scheme outlined above should be capable of answering questions concerning their responsibilities posed by the health authorities. To that end seminars should be developed to prepare personnel to appropriately respond to inquiries by an inspector. The basis of such a course should be a review of past internal and external inspection sources.

Training Records. All training should be well documented, especially GMP-related training. An individual's record should include their complete training history including internal and external courses. These records should be periodically reviewed to ensure that they are up-to-date.

13
A Regulatory Perspective

Anthony J. Trill
Principal Medicines Inspector
Medicines Control Agency
London, England

Apart from business, information, and cost-efficiency issues, many computer systems have clearly been developed in the interests of ensuring product quality and compliance with Good Manufacturing Practices (GMP), Good Laboratory Practices (GLP), and Good Clinical Practices (GCP). Benefits can be gained with automated systems such as process control, laboratory analyses, inventory control, information management systems, electronic batch records, and manufacturing execution systems. Significant commercial and product quality advantages are claimed for fully integrated manufacturing systems, embracing the entire spectrum of business and operations systems in manufacturing companies, (see Figures 13.1–13.3). This was brought home most forcefully at the First European Pharmaceutical Technology Conference, September 1993, Dusseldorf, Germany, where no less than twelve papers were presented on the subject. (1)

THE POTENTIAL BENEFITS OF NEW TECHNOLOGY

Human beings are not very good at performing repetitive tasks (such as inspection of product for errors); this can result in boredom leading

231

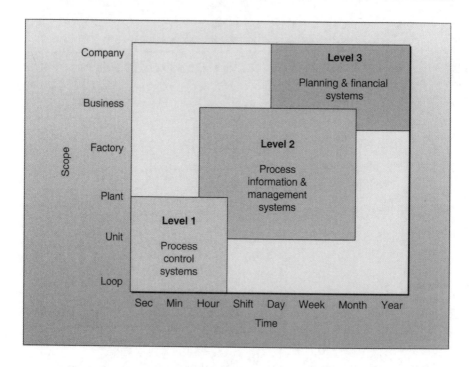

Figure 13.1. Information and operations systems. (Reproduced by kind permission of the UK PICSVF.)

to omissions and quality failures (e.g., faulty units passing inspection or transposition of numerals when copying data). (2, 3) On the other hand, robust, reliable, and responsive automated systems are ideally suited for performing simple, boring tasks accurately and reliably, resulting in zero error rates on recorded production data, and increased levels of GMP compliance at reduced cost.

With integrated systems, where connectivity difficulties have been overcome (OSI has helped here), there are also claims for reduced manufacturing cycle times, reduced waste, and more effective control over data entry and information flow. Such systems provide comprehensive system change controls and management of related change between classes of documents such as SOPs, batch masters, and so on. They also provide immediate access to information for timely decisions. (4)

During the discussion sessions at a recent European conference, a speaker concluded that with the disappearance of conventional

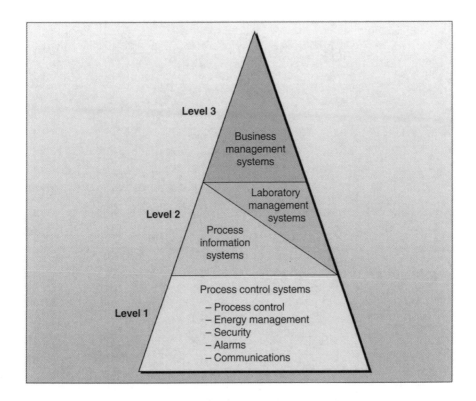

Figure 13.2. Information systems and their place in the hierarchy. (Reproduced by kind permission of the UK PICSVF.)

documents (such as manufacturing paper-based text records), object oriented techniques would be needed for verification and new auditing techniques would become necessary in place of document compliance checks. He felt this would have implications for the FDA. (5)

Having noted the advantages claimed for good quality computerized systems, it should be remembered that the process of specifying, designing, developing, and testing software relies very heavily on human ingenuity and logic. Such a process carries with it not only all the strengths but also all the weaknesses of the human psyche, from conceptual logic and design to development, implementation, and management of the live system. No one should be surprised by this potential for concern or by the interest inspectors show for evidence of good software and systems engineering practices (GSEP) in the design and quality assurance of "regulated" applications.

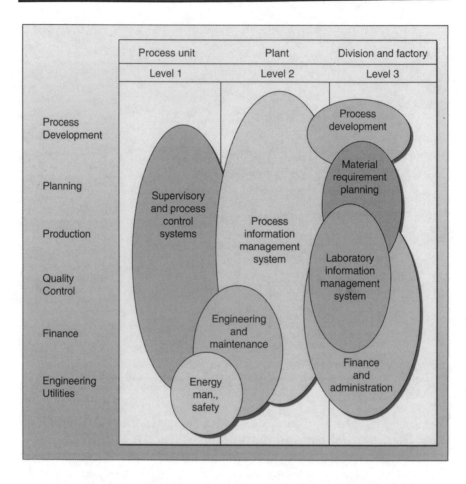

Process unit	Plant	Division and factory
Level 1	Level 2	Level 3

Process
Development

Planning

Production

Quality
Control

Finance

Engineering
Utilities

Process
development

Material
requirement
planning

Supervisory
and process
control
systems

Process
information
management
system

Laboratory
information
management
system

Engineering
and
maintenance

Energy
man.,
safety

Finance
and
administration

Figure 13.3. Integration of systems. (Reproduced by kind permission of the UK PICSVF.)

COMPUTER SYSTEMS ASSESSMENT—INSPECTOR CONCERNS

It should be remembered that the assessment of computerized systems has generally been only a small part of routine inspection work. However, with the increasing use of new technology for automation and paperless systems, more inspection time may become necessary in the future.

Inspectors are concerned with those computerized systems that have the potential to affect product quality, information, data, and security in manufacturing and other licensed operations. For example:

- Materials control applications, such as inventory control, manufacturing batch records, MRP/MRP-II, manufacturing execution systems, product distribution and recall, and so on

- Process control applications

- Entry, accuracy, integrity, security, processing, storage, durability, and retrievability of relevant data

- Computer controlled instruments, data processing, and reporting systems in laboratories and process areas

- Critical environmental control systems, or dedicated suites, such as for aseptic sterile product manufacture

- Communications and interactions with other devices and systems including networks

- Documentation control applications

When arriving on-site for an initial review of computerized operations, the author has found it useful to adopt a "top-down" approach, as illustrated in Figure 13.4, for a logical assessment of the range of systems and management arrangements, before studying particular applications in depth.

Depending on the nature and depth of the intended inspection, inspectors may consider many factors related to the design, operation, and control of regulated systems. Such factors include the following:

- Functional specifications

- The validation, control, and monitoring of the systems

- Management responsibilities, authority, and security for the systems

- Written procedures in place

- Software and equipment standards

- Records to demonstrate compliance

- Change controls

- Error and corrective action logs

- Auditing arrangements

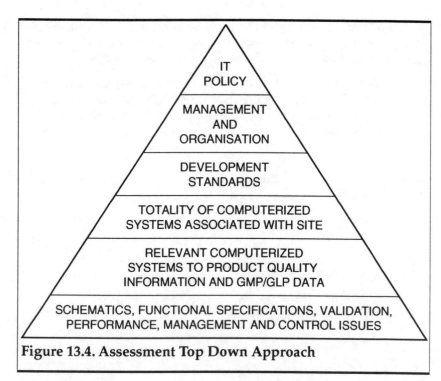

Figure 13.4. Assessment Top Down Approach

- Training

- . . . and a variety of other aspects relating to the general chapters of the EC Guide to GMP.

Detailed assessment may be necessary for some of the following elements (not intended as an exhaustive list):

- Relevant company policies and procedures for procurement, development projects, and systems management

- Descriptions of systems and interactions

- Hardware and software (user and technical support) manuals

- Key personnel in management and support

- Training arrangements for users and technical support

- Equipment—hardware and network elements and configuration

- Software-operating system (e.g., security), applications software (e.g., databases used) and other software for full functionality

- The company's assessment of Supplier's QMS and product specific project standards, quality plans, and records to support the structural testing and quality of the software

- Specifications

- Installation, Operational, and Performance Qualification

- Data handling

- Audit trails

- Error reporting and resolution

- Software and hardware maintenance procedures and records

- Backup and Disaster/Recovery arrangements

- Archiving

- Standards, Procedures, User and Technical Support Documents

- Records from Development Life Cycle, Implementation, and Running

- Demonstration of system(s)

- Physical and logical security

- Configuration management and change controls

- Auditing arrangements

These aspects, together with validation evidence, provide a measure of the accuracy and reliability of the evolving system.

Range and Interaction of Computerized Systems

Figures 13.1–13.3 serve to illustrate the potential range of computerization on sites and between sites. They take a bottom-up approach through various "levels" from level 1 through 2 and 3 to full systems integration. Level 1 comprises process control systems, energy management, security, alarms and communications; level 2, process information and laboratory information management systems; level 3, business management systems.

When information and operations systems are linked, we need to consider them on a scale from loop to company-wide activities, and from seconds to years in terms of time. As for integration, the "balloons" in Figure 13.3 suggest the degree of integration between various systems; clearly this will be a variable dependent on the nature of the company's business and operations. For integrated systems, the validation protocol needs to consider (for each separate system) the relevant programs and modules that impact on GMP and quality. Where systems have been integrated on a site (and between sites), there is in reality no totally clear boundary between systems for full functionality. Many parts of these systems may impact on GMP/GLP and product quality activities. Common sense suggests that it is important to identify which parts of the integrated systems are relevant for GMP system validation purposes in order to minimise and manage the workload.

Documentation

Documentation is necessary for every stage of system development and use to aid management, control, auditing, and inspection. In large software projects development tools are used for enforced (automatic) documentation and linking the stages. GMP and GLP guidelines also require computerized systems to be fully documented.

The primary purpose of documentation is to record and communicate to others the details of the specification, evolution, control, and characteristics of the software, hardware, and systems. The list in Table 13.1 illustrates some of the documents that are likely to be of interest to a project auditor.

Apart from comments to understand how performance is achieved, every program should incorporate records to follow decisions taken at various stages of program design, verification and eventual implementation. This helps with high level reviews and in tracing logic errors and mistakes, so that project management and controls are facilitated.

EC GMP REQUIREMENTS

The current detailed EC GMP guidelines are to be found in the latest edition of the EC Guide to GMP (now published in the UK as "Rules and Guidance for Pharmaceutical Manufacturers 1993"). (6)

This publication incorporates not only the EC Guide but also 14 annexes (Annex 11 referring specifically to Computerized Systems), EC Directives on GMP, the Code of Practice for Qualified Persons, and Standard Provisions for Manufacturer's Licences. The purpose of the Guide and annexes is to interpret the statutory "Principles and Guidelines of GMP": Directives 91/356/EEC and 91/412/EEC for Human and Veterinary Medicines, respectively. These cover a number of topics including the following, which are equally applicable to both computerized and conventional systems: Quality Management, Personnel,

Table 13.1: Audit Documentation Associated with Computer Systems Projects

- Corporate policies and procedures for project management, purchasing, developing, and controlling computer systems for "regulated" applications at all levels of complexity and life cycle stages
- Specifications for relevant systems and life cycle elements
- Audit reports on supplier's quality management systems and capabilities
- Project management standards
- Structured design methodology
- Quality plans
- Life cycle records from testing, acceptance, and ongoing operation
- Program listings
- Source code
- Programming standards and methods
- System schematics and up-to-date descriptions of the system
- Data flow charts and diagrams
- High level block diagrams
- Purpose and functionality
- Interactions and links with other systems
- Network diagrams
- Hardware and software inventories
- Operating procedures
- Training records
- User accounts
- IT Dept. (Data Centre) standards and records
- Configuration management SOPs and records
- Security (logical and physical), user access and privileges
- Specific SOPs and measures to ensure data integrity and audit trails for entry, updates or amendments of data in relevant applications
- Error referral and resolution
- Transaction logs
- Audit trails
- Change controls and linking of source, object files, and user documentation
- Commissioning and testing records
- Validation protocols and records
- Disaster/recovery arrangements
- Calibration and maintenance
- SOPs for the internal QA audit of these computer systems

Note: "Regulated" is used by the author as a global term covering GMP, GLP, GCP, GXP systems that are liable to be inspected by the appropriate regulatory or licensing bodies.

Premises and Equipment, Documentation, Production, Quality Control, Work Contracted Out, Complaints and Product Recall, and Self-Inspection. The glossary section of the Guide to GMP has definitions for "system," "computerized system," "validation," and "qualification." (See Table 13.2.)

Table 13.2: Definitions from the Glossary of the EC Guide to GMP

System   Used in the sense of a regulated pattern of interacting activities and techniques which are united to form an organized whole.

Computerized Systems   A system including the input of data, electronic processing, and the output of information to be used either for reporting or automatic control.

Validation   Action of proving, in accordance with the principles of GMP, that any procedure, process, equipment, material, activity, or system actually leads to the expected results (see also qualification).

Qualification   Action of proving that any equipment works correctly and actually leads to the expected results. The word *validation* is sometimes widened to incorporate the concept of qualification.

Article 9 of the above Directives, also known as "The GMP Directives," applies to electronic and paper-based documentation and data processing systems and states the following:

Documentation

1. The manufacturer shall have a system of documentation based upon specifications, manufacturing formulae and processing and packaging instructions, procedures and records covering the various manufacturing operations that they perform. Documents shall be clear, free from errors and kept up to date. Pre-established procedures for general manufacturing operations and conditions shall be available, together with specific documents for the manufacture of each batch. This set of documents shall make it possible to trace the history of each batch. The batch documentation shall be retained for at least one year after the expiry date of the batches to which it relates or at least five years after the certification referred to in Article 22 (2) of Directive 75/319/EEC whichever is the longer.

2. When electronic, photographic or other data processing systems are used instead of written documents, the manufacturer shall have validated the systems by proving that the data will be appropriately stored during the anticipated period of storage.

Data stored by these systems shall be made readily available in legible form. The electronically stored data shall be protected against loss or damage of data (e.g. by duplication or back-up and transfer onto another storage system).

This Article links master documents, batch related records, data processing, archiving, and retrieval systems; the requirements are equally applicable to paper-based and modern day real-time, interactive electronic batch record ("paperless") and database systems.

Chapter 4 of the Guide to GMP is concerned with Documentation and paragraph 4.9 provides amplification of Article 9 of EC Directive 91/356, by drawing attention to the need for

- Detailed procedures

- Checks on the accuracy of records

- The need for only authorised persons to be able to enter and modify data

- A record of changes and deletions

- Passwords and other restrictions and controls over access

- Second independent checks for the entry of critical data

- Specific requirements for the electronic storage and backup of batch records

It stresses the requirement for such records to be retrievable throughout the archiving period of many years, and this has implications for the hardware and operating systems platform used for retrieval (as amplified by item 13 of Annex 11).

Annex 11—Computerized Systems

The following summarizes the main requirements of Annex 11 "Computerized Systems". (For ease of reference Annex item numbers are shown in brackets after each comment for "validation" and "system" aspects): (7)

GENERAL:

Definitions (see Glossary)

Principle—refers to systems considerations, QA and compatibility issues, (e.g., with superseded systems), product quality and the need to consider principles elsewhere in the guide

Personnel issues—project and operations aspects

Validation and life cycle considerations [2]

SYSTEM:

The siting of equipment and avoidance of interference [3]

An up-to-date detailed description of the system and its interactions [4]

Software to be produced in accordance with a system of QA [5]

Running checks/validation of inputs [6]

Testing before acceptance (functional testing) [7]

Data issues: Controls, Security, Integrity [8]

Critical data: authorizations and operator identity considerations (entry, confirmation, amendment, audit trail) [9], [10]

Change controls required for system and program alterations (Revalidation, responsible persons, approval, implementation and records) [11]

It must be possible to provide hard copies of electronically stored data for quality auditing purposes [13]

Data is to be stored securely against deliberate or accidental damage (personnel, physical, electronic). Other considerations are accessibility, durability, accuracy and retrieval after proposed system changes (c.f. EC Guide 4.9 on documentation systems). [13]

Data to be protected by backing up, and stored separately [14]

Alternative arrangements need to be defined to cover breakdowns of important systems (e.g., to support recalls). [15]

Validation records are needed to cover these alternative arrangements. Records are to be kept of failures and remedies. [16]

Procedures needed for recording and analysing errors. [17]

Where outside agencies are used, a formal contract or agreement is needed with a clear statement of responsibilities (c.f. EC Guide, Chapter 7). [18]

The name of the Qualified Person effecting release of batches by computer should be recognized and recorded. [19]

PAPERLESS SYSTEMS

Companies must ensure that their thinking for the design, development, implementation, and control of integrated computerized systems takes account of the requirements of Quality Management and GMP from other parts of the EC Guide and good software engineering practices. Design and validation for such systems must also show compliance with Chapters 4, 5, 6, and 8 (Documentation, Production, Quality Control, Complaints, and Product Recall). This calls for appropriate interpretation of the terms *written* and *signed* for electronic forms of documents. Note in particular the following Paragraphs from Chapters in the Guide:

- **4.3:** authorization of documents (paper and electronic).

- **4.9:** (See p. 241).

- **4.17:** Batch Processing Record requirements, linking materials, quantities, persons, responsibilities, authorizations, equipment, times, and events.

- **4.18:** Batch Packaging Record Requirements (as for 4.17).

- **4.25:** Batch Distribution Records (to facilitate recalls).

- **4.26:** written procedures, records of actions, and conclusions for validation, equipment assembly, and calibration, and so on.

- **6.7 to 6.10:** Quality Control documentation elements, records, data handling, and original records (raw data).

- **6.15 to 6.18:** QC testing; the recording and checking of results; linking samples, specifications, references, methods procedures/events, persons, responsibilities, results, and decisions.

- **8.12 and 8.15:** distribution records and recall arrangements.

The EC Guide, Annex 11, has a specific statement on computerized systems validation in paragraph 2 and refers to life-cycle stages including software development and testing, system commissioning, documentation, operation, monitoring, and modifying. Paragraph 5 of the Annex also specifically refers to the need to ensure that the software has been produced in accordance with a system of Quality Assurance. This requires the adoption of formal QMS arrangements either in-house or at the Supplier, the assessment for compliance with such requirements and life-cycle validation evidence.

In addition to the need for quality assured software, the general GMP recommendations in the EC Guide for validation of processes, systems, procedures, and so on are equally applicable to both traditional and computerized systems.

Paragraphs 5.21 to 5.24 cover the conduct of validation work, records, process considerations, and re-validation.

QUALITY ASSURANCE OF SOFTWARE AND SYSTEMS PROJECTS

To design, develop, coordinate, install, implement, and use successfully any new computer system, whether it has been produced in-house or purchased, requires effective project management. The three principal activities associated with project management are planning, controlling, and monitoring. A successful project requires sound plans and procedures, and a responsible and visible project management team that will exercise firm control in an organisation matched to the project's needs.

Areas of Concern

Within the limits of its host hardware, software can satisfy a great variety of user requirements, and incorporate customised facilities tailored in fine detail. However, software development can be difficult to control, partly because users think it is so easy to change facilities and underestimate the technical complexity of proposed changes and developments. Projects incorporating a large complex software component require special management attention to

- Establish a clear and detailed statement of user requirements and acceptance test criteria
- Assess the quality assurance systems employed by possible suppliers
- Establish a mechanism for controlling change
- Monitor compliance, progress, and quality

The purchaser's project manager may find it difficult to keep the project under control unless adequate requests for compliance with requirements are included in the tender document. It is important to seek compliance on any aspects of the project (user and technical requirements, methods of working, purchaser/supplier interfaces, arrangements for maintenance, training, and support, etc.) which will require supplier resource and cooperation.

This author has noted that successful pharmaceutical companies often establish multidisciplinary technical project teams to control and coordinate the introduction of new technology and the associated quality assurance measures. These teams are increasingly interested in the specification, validation, and auditing of computer systems in licensable operations.

Best Practices

Due to the iterative nature of software development and the interdependence of programs and modules in interactive systems, it is not often possible to demonstrate software QA simply by testing the functionality of the finished product.

Quality has to be demonstrably built into such software. Project controls, quality plans, and formal methods are required for specifications, design, development, coding, testing, modifications/change control, and implementation, with documented records throughout to provide evidence of structural quality for validation purposes. Project management tools (e.g., PRINCE) (8), system design methodologies (e.g., SSADM) (9), and institutions such as the National Measurement Accreditation Service (NAMAS) (10) assist in this process.

Within the EC GMP guidelines there is room for interpretation and the evolution of "Best Practices". Some of these best practices are considered in recent articles published in *Pharmaceutical Technology International*. (11) See also Table 13.3, which provides a brief summary.

SDLC Approach

A prerequisite to ensuring the control and management of software and systems projects is the adoption of a system development life cycle (SDLC) model, with strict configuration management and change controls. (The Annex 11 validation statement refers to a life cycle concept). STARTS literature from the National Computing Centre, Manchester, England (12), provides such models and techniques and the U.S. PMA have published a version showing flow charts for new and existing systems. (13) These SDLCs fit well with international standards and

Table 13.3: Quality and Project Management Best Practices for Purchasers of Pharmaceutical Computerized Systems

1. Ensure that the management of IT systems, projects, and support is clearly defined.

2. Take a top-down approach in setting and applying corporate policies and standards to the procurement and operational aspects of IT and automation systems.

3. Apply a recognized system development life cycle model (SDLC) and ensure full validation documentation and controls.

4. Project teams to set standards and establish quality and project plans based on Good Software Engineering Practice (GSEP).

5. Adopt International or National standards where possible.

6. Assess the QMS of potential suppliers and the quality of proprietary items.

7. Favour suppliers certified to quality standards such as TickIT, EN29001-3, ISO 9000-3, STARTS, and assess relevance of certification.

8. Insist on structured quality methodologies, full records, and change controls at suppliers/contractors.

9. Place formal strict contracts. Cover all technical, quality issues, and deliverables.

10. Qualify and validate the systems. Formalise acceptance reports, handover, and signing off.

11. Continue to control and document the systems to SDLC.

12. Ensure ongoing monitoring and auditing of the systems for compliance with GMP and Good IT Practices (GITP). Consider configuration management, audit trails, security, data integrity, and change controls over system data and records.

Good Software and System Engineering Practices (GSEP). The "VMAN" and Good Automated Manufacturing Practice (GAMP) validation initiatives from the UK PICSVF (see later in this chapter) also make use of a life cycle project and quality management concept. Examples of the various SDLC models are shown in Figures 13.5–13.8.

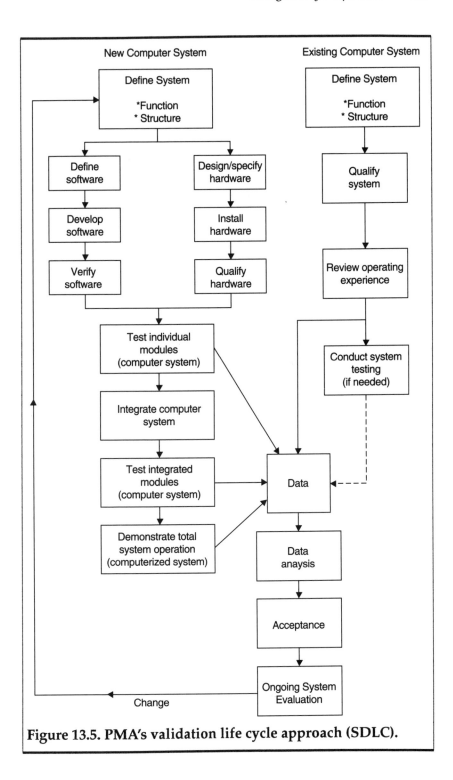

Figure 13.5. PMA's validation life cycle approach (SDLC).

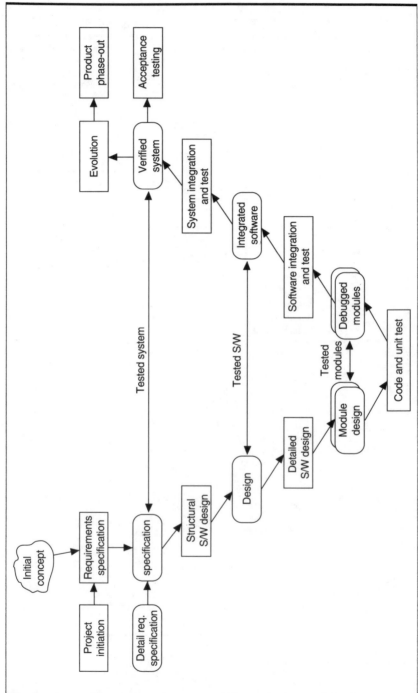

Figure 13.6. Life cycle schematic: life cycle V model. (From STARTS Publications, National Computing Centre, Ltd., Oxford Road, Manchester, M1 7ED.)

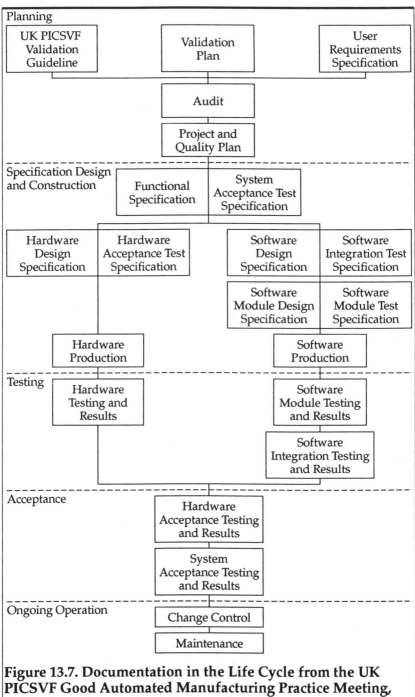

Figure 13.7. Documentation in the Life Cycle from the UK PICSVF Good Automated Manufacturing Practice Meeting, Validation of Automated Systems in Pharmaceutical Manufacture, Guideline, London, 1994. (with permission of UK PICSVF)

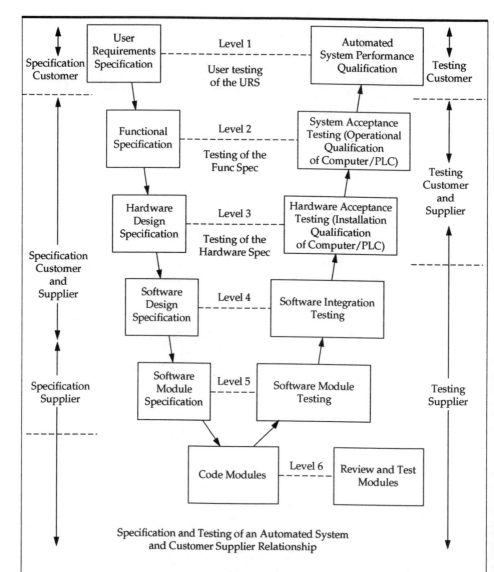

Figure 13.8. V-model showing Customer-Supplier Relationship During Specification and Testing from UK PICSVF Good Automated Manufacturing Practice Meeting, Validation of Automated Systems in Pharmaceutical Manufacture Guideline, London, 1994. (with permission of UK PICSVF)

SOFTWARE CERTIFICATION

With proprietary software packages and for bespoke work, the certification of a software supplier's Quality Management System and products by approved assessors may offer a way forward. (14) The application of GSEP, together with comprehensive verification and validation arrangements, strict configuration management, and change controls, is essential.

GSEP Approach

GSEP ensures that there is a project plan covering the intended implementation of the system together with a quality plan defining the standards to be applied to all products (i.e., "deliverables" from each development stage), and the verification and validation arrangements to be used to demonstrate and record that they are acceptable. The quality plan should include an audit trail for the project, clearly demonstrating the traceabilty of requirements through to the solution.

GSEP ensures that there is an authorized written statement of requirements which will ultimately be used as the basis of the customer's validation of the system's correct performance, together with an authorized written validation protocol defined by, or with the agreement of, the user. This protocol will be used to demonstrate that the system meets functional requirements. On installation the supplier may be able to apply GSEP standard techniques and tools to analyse, implement, and test the system, resulting in a well-engineered system that is easy to maintain.

Test Plans and Ongoing Control

Test plans to demonstrate inputs, processing, and outputs require a great deal of thought and should include data precision, the maintenance of raw data, security, and audit trails. The results of all testing and modification work must be formally recorded together with signed acceptance for the customer/user.

Following acceptance, the purchasers need to control the documented system, ensuring that modification proposals and changes re-enter the iterative scheme of the system development life cycle model. An on-going means of monitoring and auditing the system should be established to ensure compliance with GMP and good IT practices.

VALIDATION OF EXISTING SYSTEMS

A number of older existing systems have not been fully validated and documented as they have evolved over the years. Many of these are fairly complex and some firms have expressed concern about how to meet GMP requirements.

There is nothing new in the requirement for validated systems to be in place, yet a number of companies find that they do not even have up-to-date descriptions of their systems as required by Annex 11 (4) of the EC Guide, let alone evidence relating to software quality or validation.

Where the system has a direct impact on product quality and patient safety, then the age of the system cannot be used as an excuse for not meeting standards. Firms often claim that solutions are not always readily apparent, either due to proprietary factors or a multitude of evolved in-house programs with no clear database management system. One thing is certain, however; unlike a vintage wine, software will not improve simply with ageing.

Certainly with existing complex business and information systems (e.g., production batch control, MRP/MRP-II), my experience confirms that life cycle documentation, from requirements/design specification through all the subsequent development, testing, and implementation phases is unlikely to be complete or available. The issue is complicated by the use of underlying proprietary core database software and the configuration work to tailor the package for the pharmaceutical application.

For information and business package systems, it is difficult to obtain data on proprietary software unless there is supplier cooperation. It is unlikely to be either feasible or cost-effective to reverse engineer a large proprietary database system (for example). Other measures of the quality of the underlying software are required together with full validation of the configured (or tailored) aspects of the package.

Table 13.4 seeks to give an example of how to approach the retrospective documentation of "Support Systems" where (regulated) configured application programs are installed to support manufacturing and quality control (business and information levels). This is one possible approach to contain the documentation and retrospective validation effort for underlying supporting hardware and software. It should ideally be supplemented with a supplier/vendor quality assessment audit, or certification reports and commentary from experienced users and support staff on the currency and value of the documentation.

Full controls, QA, and documentation is, however, possible for the user's configuration of the proprietary package and this needs to be undertaken in depth.

Table 13.4: Retrospective Documentation of Hardware and Software Support Systems for a Configured Application Running at "ABC" Company

1. Identify the specific hardware and software elements required for validated operation of the Application Software at ABC Company. These form the "Support System" for the Configured Application.

    *   Hardware configuration including class of computer, make and model

    *   System Hardware Concepts (e.g., machine architecture, data storage and retrieval, CPU/microprocessor hierarchy)

    *   System Software Concepts (e.g., operating system, executive software, configuration software, database arrangements, communications, security module, etc.)

    *   Network configuration and security management

    *   Other installed software for specific functions, such as data entry, remote transmissions, or database queries

2. Compile a written inventory of all documentation associated with the Support System hosting the Configured Application at ABC Company today, including supplier manuals, IT Management, and support documentation.

    *   Service contracts

    *   Vendor hardware and software product manuals

    *   System logbooks or alternative system change control records

    *   License version control records

    *   Maintenance and support records

    *   Upgrade and new version installation records (e.g., arrangements for release, version, and system changes)

    *   Data centre (IT Dept.) policies and procedures for systems management, such as

        —Configuration management

        —System backup & disaster recovery

        —Data archiving procedure

        —Physical and logical security policies

        —Personnel training and experience records

3. Use the above documents to establish a timeline of significant events in the life of the Support System hosting the Configured Application at ABC Company today.

Continued on next page

Table 13.4 continued

4. Write a report on the way Support System hardware and software elements are used by the regulated Configured Application being validated.

    *   Which modules are reliant on Support System performance?

    *   How are priviledges (access and authority) to Configured Application and Support System given and monitored?

    *   Describe today's configuration.

    —Hardware and software versions

    —Data centre/IT Dept and service relationship

    —Manufacturing/QC structures and functions using the Configured Application

    —Role of key users: what parts of the system they use and for what purposes such as relational database priviledges or other access

    —Training available for new Support System staff

    —Software and hardware maintenance procedures

    —Disaster recovery and backup procedures

    —Documentation listing: SOPs available, product manuals, operations manuals, and so on

    —Support System vendor contractual arrangements for support and enhancements: hardware, software, service, networks

    —Any recent audit findings

5. Use a Signature Page to record Manufacturing and QA review and approval of the current report.

6. Include an author('s) page with signatures and brief CV of relevant experience that qualifies them to know what they have written about the Support System.

Satisfactory evidence from second and third party audits, appropriate quality system certification (such as TickIT) of the vendor/developer plus product specific benchmark testing, and evidence from a large number of purchasers helps to build confidence in the underlying software package. Good quality documentation and version control from the supplier and developer is essential. Accuracy, reliability, data integrity (security), and audit trail issues are all important in these data handling sytems.

Evaluating Older Systems

Some business and information systems may have been in use in pharmaceutical companies for a number of years. An effort has to be made to judge their quality and attempt to limit the extent of any retrospective validation work. It is sensible for knowledgeable users to discuss and report on experiences with existing systems in a working party structure, to identify strengths and weaknesses, and to consider performance measures for each system.

Change controls need to be established immediately (if they are lacking). Areas of concern should be identified together with status reports on upstream documentation elements that would normally support the system development life cycle. It is possible that independent system software may also assist in reporting on the operating characteristics of the application programs, especially where there is little by way of documented operational history. Vendor supplied documents should also be considered for standard purchased proprietary systems.

If the working party expresses confidence in the system(s) after the review process, then project management and validation arrangements should be set in train, working to accepted validation and verification procedures to define the validation plan, test plans, and documentation effort to re-qualify the system in the operational and maintenance phase of its life cycle. The author has noted that some companies have been able to limit testing to exceptions and boundaries only (for some systems), where justified by good operating experience and quality measures.

A system history, compiled by staff with the most experience operating the system is a useful document. It should provide a description of the system—its functional specification—and refer to documents linking the original procurement proposal, acceptance testing, system and user manuals and records, maintenance, upgrades, code modifications, and audit reports. Additional reports are also needed to confirm user experiences with the system and to confirm the present arrangements for configuration, authorised use, and system assurance measures for the system (e.g., backup, disaster/recovery, security, data controls and authorised users, training, version control, software maintenance, support documentation lists, contractual support arrangements, audits, etc.). Those retrospective documents will hopefully provide evidence of the compliance of the system.

This retrospective definition and documentation of the system as to function, structure, user accounts, security, and access controls (with any redundant code either having been removed or isolated), together with the verification and testing work provides requalification evidence. After this the system should continue to be subject to full change control procedures and configuration management to ensure that only authorised changes are implemented for user requirements, code, system, screen formats, reports, and so on. (Future code changes, testing, and approval should ideally take place away from the "live" production system with controlled release ultimately to the user environment.)

As with forward (life cycle) validation work, users should be involved in establishing the validation test protocols (and acceptance criteria) for the analysis of data generated from functional testing. There should be full documentation with signed reasoning and approvals throughout.

Thereafter, performance of the system should be routinely monitored and evaluated, with consideration also given to the various runtime transaction logs, error logs, audit trails, and exception reports that may be required to demonstrate the accuracy and reliability of the system.

CRITICAL APPLICATIONS

Certainly, both the control and monitoring systems for high risk applications (such as autoclaves, freeze driers, and other Level 1 programmable process control applications supporting sterile product processes) must be documented, quality assured, and validated as they have a direct impact on product quality and patient safety.

Reverse Engineering

Reverse engineering is an option to consider when the system is of a critical nature and there is no other way of obtaining detailed information and documentation on the development and quality status of the software. Where both compiled executable code and source code have been supplied with the system, then proprietary development tools may be used to carry out a variety of tests on code whilst it is running, to undertake debugging and to provide documentation on the control logic and the technical description of the program.

The amount of retrospective work that may be necessary will be dictated by the particular process control application, the state of archived software project life cycle records (if any), and a review of operating experience. For example, the absence of approved functional specifications and a lack of commented code and testing records (e.g., variables and arrays, input and output verification, boundary testing, critical algorithms, procedures, set points, sensor failures, error messages and alarms, etc.) makes the retrospective work more demanding.

Ultimately, for systems regarded as high risk (such as automated sterilizers—Level 1 process control), then companies must be able to demonstrate the use of professionally written, validated control software and validated monitoring arrangements. The author's inspection experience has confirmed that reverse engineering has been used successfully for a series of large computer controlled autoclaves where the software developer has been unable to supply the necessary life cycle and quality assurance documentation for the software.

Integration

Automated manufacturing applications bring together the products and components of an expanding variety of disciplines, applied sciences, and technologies. Considerable expertise is often called for to provide the advanced electronic, mechanical, systems, and software engineering solutions demanded by the project specifications; not surprisingly, very few pharmaceutical companies have this expertise in-house. It is noted that service companies specialising in systems integration are being used increasingly by the pharmaceutical industry to provide the multidisciplinary expertise necessary to ensure the satisfactory completion of large projects. Systems integrators have often worked on demanding projects in other regulated industry sectors (such as aerospace, defence, nuclear, banking, etc.). Solutions to apparently difficult issues may be more readily achieved by applying tried and tested techniques from other industries, thus minimising costs, avoiding the "reinvention of the wheel", and containing risks.

Logic Controllers

Programmable logic controllers have to be documented, validated, and controlled like any other computer system, with the software (e.g., ladder logic) version controlled and placed under configuration management.

Proportional-Integral-Derivative Controllers (PID) should be documented and controlled through tuning and calibration (e.g., zero and span) and performance testing (verifying input signal to device performance), inputs/outputs qualified from simulation, and full functional acceptance testing. Loop specifications and systems configuration databases must be defined, tested, and subjected to change control.

It is also important to define and control any system configurable parameters and variable switch settings, associated with the process control equipment, that can vary such functions as "high/low limits", "range", "enable", "disable", "alarms", and so on to avoid invalid control sequences during the product process, and the possibility of disastrous results or lost batches of product.

Hard-wired links (e.g., safety critical) should be defined and tested separately and as part of the integrated system.

Automation

As discussed earlier in this chapter, human beings are not very good at performing repetitive tasks requiring prolonged concentration as this can lead to boredom and the introduction of errors. The case is often made for robust, reliable, and responsive automated systems being ideally suited to performing such simple, repetitive boring tasks accurately and reliably.

The automation of manufacturing, control, and support systems is gathering momentum and seems to be inexorable. Integrated systems are said to offer not only the potential for improved levels of GMP compliance and cost savings, but also the provision of effective and efficient controls over data and information. Claims are also made for the electronic management, linking, and version control of all "documentation", including SOPs, batch masters, labels, leaflets, and so on, thus reducing opportunities for errors.

PACKAGING LINE APPLICATIONS

In the first ten months of 1993, 21 percent of defect reports to the MCA Medicinal Products Defect Report Centre in London were related to label, printing, or filling defects. These concerned incorrect products in containers, missing labels, incorrect labels, incorrect strengths or instructions, and significant errors in label text. We continue to experience significant product quality problems relating to faulty product packaging operations; these often result not only in defect reports but also drug alert letters and recalls from the marketplace. If proper control and detection systems were in place at both the printed component suppliers and on the pharmaceutical companies packaging lines, then it should be possible to reduce the incidence of these defects quite substantially.

With certain packaging line security systems, reliance has been placed on performance validation and the use of validated, fail-safe, independent monitoring either downstream or in parallel with the system or device, measuring the same or alternative relevant parameters, building in some redundancy. This may be a justifiable approach, where, for example there is little or no supplier cooperation regarding the proprietary software. This must be supported with full acceptance testing for functionality, calibration, correct maintenance, and control of the primary computerized device and routine challenge testing.

Computerized equipment used in Packaging Departments must be reliable and qualified in respect of its performance. Reasonable measures are needed to ensure that the software has been produced in a quality assured manner and that specification, design, coding, and testing life cycle elements can be traced if necessary. It is for the pharmaceutical users to satisfy themselves that the systems are robust, reliable, responsive, and adequately documented and supported.

Clearly for "stand-alone" instruments of limited variability on packing lines, calibration, acceptance testing, subsequent controls, and parametric checks or challenges may well be sufficient.

However, where on-line instruments are either programmable or manipulating data, carrying out SPC (Statistical Process Control) and producing reports (such as on some sophisticated check-weighers, etc.) or where linked to other supervisory and control systems (controlling or acquiring data), then more detailed validation protocols are required to verify the integrated functionality and also the key algorithms, set points, alarms, error messages, control and failure logic, and so on. There should also be an assessment of the supplier's controls over the quality of the software. At the very least certificated sets of test results from software structural testing should be made available. These should demonstrate compliance with specifications. For new systems full forward life-cycle validation is the most efficient approach.

It may be salutary to recall that paragraph 4.26 of the EC Guide indicates that there should be written procedures and associated records, for validation, equipment assembly and calibration, maintenance, and training. Inspectors will expect to see these procedures and records in respect of Computerized Systems.

DATABASE PACKAGES AND INTEGRATED SYSTEMS

Proprietary database packages and integrated systems present a challenge. One option proposed for the future is for underlying software QA to be certified to relevant international standards (by auditing and testing). Purchasers would then be sold certified licensed replicate copies of the package(s), together with full supporting documentation for configuration, use, and maintenance. The purchaser/user, in configuring the proprietary packages would be expected (as now), to exercise full life-cycle, project, and quality management controls over the specifications and records (e.g., user requirements, function, design, development, coding, testing, acceptance, and on-going operation) in respect of the configured application programs and data handling. We are already seeing substantial progress towards meeting the first part, with many suppliers obtaining certification to TickIT to the software-sector specific QA assessment schedules in ISO 9000-3.

Users should ensure that their configured application packages are fully documented and controlled in accordance with Good Software Engineering Practices and meet the requirements of the GMP guidelines.

For new projects a controlled sequence of events to a SDLC model approach, fully documented to GMP requirements, is required for all systems.

In the author's experience the most successful companies have ensured through training and/or recruitment a minimum level of expertise and competence in understanding and controlling computerized systems within technical management in QA and Production. These people are essential for an effective dialogue with the IT Department, vendors, project managers, consultants, and inspectors.

Ultimately, it is for named responsible persons on licences to consider particular computerized system applications and come to a reasoned judgement on the adequacy of documentation and validation evidence. They should be prepared to explain and justify these matters to Inspectors.

EVIDENCE OF STRUCTURED QUALITY SYSTEMS

Standard methodologies and tools force developers to adopt controlled techniques and disciplines for tasks and documentation. This, in turn, provides evidence for the purchaser, to support the functional accuracy and reliability claims for the resulting system, (e.g., PRINCE; SSADM; CASE tools; TickIT; and relevant EN, ISO, IEEE/ANSI, IEE, BS, and DIN standards).

For a number of years pharmaceutical companies have been encouraged to audit the Quality Management Systems used by manufacturers who supply their starting materials and components to ensure that they meet acceptable standards. The Quality Management Systems used by their application software suppliers should likewise be audited. Pharmaceutical companies can also seek the assessment and certification of vendors by recognised standards bodies to current

ISO 9000 Quality Standards and assessment schedules, but until recently there has not been a pharmaceutical sector specific scheme. (15) (22)

The UK's Department of Trade and Industry's (DTI) policy has been to encourage independent third-party testing and certification, and this has generated a growing interest in the EC. The European Committee for IT Certification (ECITC) was set up, with the task of coordinating national actions and ensuring compatibility and mutual recognition of certificates. It is important that well-established National Certification Schemes provide equivalent confidence levels and that certificates are mutually recognised.

Within "TickIT", ISO 9000-3 provides guidelines for the application of ISO 9001, the international quality system standard, to software. The guidelines provide the necessary disciplines for developing quality software and importantly in a GMP/GLP context, producing the evidence (records and documents) of the checks and controls that were applied during the development of the software and its subsequent validation.

Note: It is important to recognize the superiority of the TickIT certification scheme over "generic" ISO 9001. Unlike the latter, TickIT is based on sector specific guidance in ISO 9000-3 and the use of *approved* auditors and *accredited* certification bodies. Auditor-technical compliance and the scope of certification are important. These issues are also addressed by the DISC "TickIT" executive. (14)

Software Quality Management Standards

In April 1988 the European Organisation for Quality (EOQC) held a multinational conference, entitled "First European Seminar on Software Quality", in Brussels. (16)

In the same month Logica published a DTI-sponsored report on Quality Management Standards for Software (QMSs). (17). Part of their brief had been to examine the possibility of harmonising military and civil standards. With reservations, they concluded that ISO 9001 was the best way forward for QMSs. Weaknesses were identified in the areas of total quality management, control of design iteration, configuration management, verification of tools for design purposes, and quality costs. Price-Waterhouse also reported to DTI at that time on the costs and benefits of software quality standards, indicating that the purchaser was bearing a significant cost in maintaining and correcting poor quality purchased software. (18)

The Logica report favoured third-party assessment by competent authorities, but expressed concern over the current qualifications, training, and experience of personnel involved in assessing QMSs for software.

Then, in 1989 the British Computer Society reported for DTI on a study to define a Software Sector Certification Scheme. This outlined a scheme for the organisation, procedures, mechanisms, and rules leading to the assessment and certification of software quality management systems to ISO 9001. During this period working groups were set up to study Guidance Material and requirements for auditors and lead assessors. Their recommendations have recently been adopted and promoted as the "TickIT" Guide. (19)

TickIT Guide and Certification Bodies

The guidance (172 pages of text) relates to the construction and formal assessment of software QMSs for certification to the requirements of ISO 9001 *through the application of ISO 9000-3 guidance* within the TickIT scheme. The guide has been produced to align with evolving directives of the EC and European IT sector agreement group. First published in 1990 with an updated version in 1992, the document has the following structure:

Part 1: Introduction

An introduction to certification, quality management issues, and a brief overview of ISO 9001. The text is drawn from a number of sources including "Preparing Documented Quality Systems", produced by BSI QA.

Part 2: ISO 9000-3 Guidelines for the Application of ISO 9001 to the Development Supply and Maintenance of Software

An authoritative interpretation of what the requirements set out in ISO 9001 mean in the production of information systems and products which involve software development.

Part 3: Purchaser's Guide

An explanation of the purchaser's expectations of a supplier's QMS assessed and certified to ISO 9001. This section is a précis of chapter 5 of the STARTS Purchaser's Handbook.

Part 4: Supplier's Guide

Guidance for suppliers and in-house developers implementing quality management systems for compliance to ISO 9001. This section is based on the UK's Computing Services Association's QA Working Paper on quality systems, supplemented by material from chapter 2F of the STARTS Guide.

Part 5: Auditor's Guide

Guidance for auditors on methods of conducting assessments of suppliers seeking certification of their QMS to ISO 9001. This part includes the European IT Quality System Auditor Guide which has been produced by European IT certification bodies and representatives from the IT industry with support from the Commission of the European Communities. The guide provides a common basis for auditor enquiries and facilitates audit consistency and depth of enquiry.

The guide does not pretend to provide an answer to all the problems of implementing a QMS. Specific business environments and special application issues, such as safety critical systems, impose additional requirements.

BSI Quality Assurance, Bureau Veritas Quality International Ltd, Det norske Veritas Quality Assurance, Lloyd's Register Quality Assurance, and SGS Yarsley Quality Assured Firms are TickIT-accredited certification bodies. Enquiries concerning the TickIT scheme may be addressed either to one of the certification bodies or to the DISC TickIT Office, 2 Park Street, London W1A 2BS (Tel:+44(0)71 602 8536/Fax:+44(0)71 602 8912). As of 1 May 1993 the TickIT scheme came under the auspices of DISC (Delivering Information Solutions to Customers through International Standards). DISC was established within the British Standards Institution with the support of industry and government. The TickIT Guide (ISBN 0-9519309-0-7) Issue 2, price £25.00, is available from the DISC Office, together with a newsletter, case studies, and listings of TickIT certificated firms. There are now many hundreds of firms, spanning the globe, that are certificated under this scheme.

Standards Support from EC Directives

Directive 83/189/EEC (as amended by Directive 88/182/EEC) outlined procedures for the provision of technical standards and regulations, and the exchange of information in the EC. The text for these is included in Volume 1 of "The Rules Governing Medicinal Products in the European Community" (Updated edition 1992). This document provides definitions of terms and states mechanisms for communication within the EC on technical matters. It also lists the standards institutions by name and address in the respective EC member states.

UK Pharmaceutical Industry Computer Systems Validation Forum (PICSVF) and Good Automated Manufacturing Practice (GAMP)

This group, formed in 1990/1991, had the task of improving industry's understanding of regulations for computerized systems and sought to improve communications on these issues not only within the pharmaceutical industry but also with its suppliers.

VMAN

The Forum piloted prototypes of its Validation Management paper (VMAN–II) and consulted with the industry in 1992/93. The working drafts of the VMAN documents and case studies were discussed at several seminars (20), and referenced in *Pharmaceutical Technology International*. (21)

The guidelines seek to formalise the project methodology and contractual terms for new systems between a customer and a supplier, specifying the management system, documentation, and records for subsequent acceptance by the customer.

The proposals cover responsibilities, supplier audits, quality plans, project plans, life cycle activities (specifications for all stages), production, testing, acceptance, maintenance, documented design reviews, controls over software/documents/changes and subcontractors, and training requirements. The document is supported by many detailed appendices from an SOP for Vendor Audits, through Procedures for Specifications for all Life Cycle stages to testing, the issue of software, documentation, and change controls.

GAMP

The current version of the guidelines, "Validation of Automated Systems in Pharmaceutical Manufacturing", was approved by the Forum in January 1994. This document was formally launched at a conference entitled "Good Automated Manufacturing Practice in the Pharmaceutical Industry" (GAMP) held in London on 1 March 1994, and organised by Management Forum Ltd. (22) (See also Figures 13.7 and 13.8.)

The conference was aimed at promoting discussion and consensus within the pharmaceutical business (Suppliers, Purshasers, Developers, and Users) and regulatory bodies about what represents good automated manufacturing practice in the mid-1990s. The meeting was chaired by Mr. B. H. Hartley (Chief Pharmacist, Dept. of Health, UK, and Head of Inspection and Enforcement at the Medicines Control

Agency) and speakers included David Selby (Glaxo Manufacturing Services), Anthony Trill (MCA), Ken Chapman (Pfizer Inc. USA), Anthony Margetts (Zeneca Pharmaceuticals), Robert Newton (SAL-Southtrim Autoclaves), Nick Townsend (Beckman Instruments), Richard Weirich (SAP), Graham Cassford (Logica Industry Ltd), Peter Evans (Fisons Pharmaceuticals Ltd), Sion Wyn (FJ Systems Ltd), and Paul Hewlett (NACCB, DTI). Following the conference it is intended that there will be a consultation period for feedback and comment on the guidelines from purchasers, suppliers, regulators, integrators, trade associations, and other interested parties. These comments will be considered by the PICSVF with a view to incorporating them in the final document, due to be published in January 1995 by Logica Industry Ltd for the PICSVF.

The meeting was well attended and participants agreed that it was a "Landmark Event", pointing the way ahead. It was hoped that the Guideline would ultimately have wide acceptance by industry and the accredited certification bodies. To achieve this would require "ownership" and an executive authority.

The NACCB (National Accreditation Council for Certification Bodies) have recently supported an aeronautical sector scheme and the IQA/PQG (Institute of Quality Assurance/Pharmaceutical Quality Group) have guidelines to support the assessment and certification of suppliers of starting materials to the pharmaceutical industry.

TickIT Plus GAMP

The TickIT (ISO 9000-3 assessed) supplier QMS certification initiative compliments the product (and process capability) related GAMP validation guideline. Together they provide a framework, understanding, and measure of the requirements, standards, models, methods, controls, and documentation necessary to ensure good quality software and systems, meeting performance requirements *for the pharmaceutical sector*. The Good Automated Manufacturing Practice guidelines will provide much needed additional guidance as to how to ensure that new systems comply with FDA and EC Guide *validation* requirements.

The GAMP guideline builds on recognised published standards and best practices in the various disciplines, in a commonsense fashion, demonstrating life cycle quality assurance and validation. The high quality of the guideline launched in London in March 1994 is due in no small measure to a cooperative approach taken by suppliers, the pharmaceutcal industry, system integrators, and the regulators. This is to be applauded.

The guideline could play an important role on the supply side by assisting in establishing clear requirements with vendors, some of whom have expressed a lack of appreciation of requirements for computerized systems for the pharmaceutical industry. It should also simplify project management, commissioning, and validation for the purchasers. It should reduce the time and costs spent auditing and advising suppliers and result in good quality products, documented, and validated to meet the requirements of the pharmaceutical industry and the regulatory bodies. For the suppliers it should result in a reduced validation effort for subsequent versions (replicates) of validated products.

PREPARING FOR AN INSPECTION

Computerized systems of GMP/GLP significance have been inspected as part of routine inspections, by the Department of Health/MCA, since the mid-1970s. In recent years the degree of computerization on-site has increased significantly and more detailed inspections are sometimes necessary. Companies are expected to be familiar with the relevant GMP requirements and to have reviewed and documented their systems. Initial visits to sites will often take a top-down approach to gain an overview of the range of computer applications on-site and the relevant standards and documentation in place. Particular applications are then more readily followed up in detail. Table 13.5 indicates the sort of information that should be made readily available by companies for inspectors at an early stage.

Table 13.5: Preparing for an Inspection

Ensure that the following information can be made available, if necessary, for review by the inspector:

Overview/General

1 Details of the organisation and management of IT/Computer Services and Project Engineering on-site.

2. The corporate policies on procurement of hardware, software, and systems for use in GMP/GLP areas.

3. A list of IT/Computer Services Standards and SOPs.

Continued on next page

Table 13.5 continued

4. The project management standards and procedures that have been applied to the development of the various applications.

5. Identify work contracted out routinely for systems support and maintenance.

6. A list of all Computerized Systems on-site by name and application for business, management, information, and automation levels (include basic schematics of installed hardware and networks).

More Detail on Relevant Systems

7. Identify and list those systems, subsystems, modules, and/or programs that are relevant to GMP/GLP and product quality (cross-refer to the lists provided for "6" above).

8. Provide details of disaster-recovery, backup, change controls, and configuration management.

9. A summary of documentation that generally exists to provide up-to-date descriptions of the systems and to show physical arrangements, data flows, interactions with other systems, and life cycle and validation records. The summary should indicate whether all of these systems have been fully documented and validated.

10. A statement on the qualifications and training background of personnel engaged in design, coding, testing, validation, installation, and operation of computerized systems (including consultants and subcontractors) (Specifications, Job descriptions, Training logs).

11. State the firm's approach to assessing potential suppliers of hardware, software, and systems.

12. Specify how the firm determines whether purchased or "in-house" software has been produced in accordance with a system of QA and how validation work is undertaken.

13. Document the approach that is taken to the validation and documentation of older systems where original records are inadequate.

14. Summarise the significant computer system changes made since the last inspection and plans for future developments.

15. Ensure that records relating to the various systems are readily available, well organized, and key staff are prepared to present, discuss, and review the detail, as necessary.

Note: Items 8 to 15 refer to those systems and elements identified in response to item 7.

CONCLUSIONS

This chapter has considered the following:

- The benefits and weaknesses associated with computerized systems

- The range and extent of systems interaction, illustrating the complex issues relating to full functionality, documentation, change control, and validation

- The legitimate concerns of inspectors in the context of GMP/GLP.

- Summaries of relevant EC GMP guidance and definitions

- The importance of demonstrating the quality assurance of software

- Project management issues and best practices to ensure that quality is built into software and systems

- The importance of the life cycle model

- Sector quality management systems, auditing, and certification schemes (Quality Standards and ISO 9000-3; EN29001-TickIT, etc.)

- Good Software and Systems Engineering Practice

- Existing sytems and retrospective work, where documentation is inadequate

- The GAMP initiative to establish consensus guidelines for good *automated* manufacturing practice (UK PICSVF)

- Preparing for an inspection

It is concluded that systems with the potential to affect quality should be clearly defined, documented, and validated with the need to appreciate the different development issues, skills, standards, validation requirements, and operational control/security features, depending on the "level", specific application, and risk assessment.

Where there is a clear information services strategy, defining application needs and priorities, there is the opportunity to ensure that effective, efficient, integrated systems are installed. This is achieved through the application of relevant, well-controlled and documented information technology with the necessary infrastructure and services. Such an approach should help to ensure in-built quality and compliance with GMP as well as business strategies.

For systems wholly or partly purchased from a supplier, the purchaser needs a comprehensive measure (whether by direct assessment or third-party certification such as TickIT EN29001) of the Quality Management Systems used by suppliers and to formally agree with the supplier's necessary quality and project controls to achieve a validated pharmaceutical system. Change controls, disaster/recovery, configuration management, security arrangements, and audit trails are fundamental.

Global challenges for the future will surely include the recognition of sector-based international quality management standards, together with certification arrangements for suppliers and developers to these standards, for equipment and systems. There have been apparent difficulties in the USA and a lack of confidence due to the use of *generic* ISO 9000 certification, which bears no relation to the sector specific accredited TickIT scheme. The TickIT (ISO 9000-3) and GAMP guideline initiatives are very important here. Their adoption should actually improve quality whilst reducing the number of direct assessments carried out by purchasers on prospective suppliers, resulting in cost savings from fewer QMS audits and lower maintenance/recovery costs for purchased systems. Purchasers and suppliers would have a better understanding of each other's terms of reference; for specific projects both parties would then be able to target resources on project management, design, quality, validation, and performance issues for specific software/computer systems products.

For the future, further working party initiatives on risk assessment and retrospective work would seem to be indicated, to establish best practices and to contain the workload.

ACKNOWLEDGEMENTS

Some parts of this chapter, including figures 13.1–13.5 are based on articles published by the author in *Pharmaceutical Technology International.* (23) The author would like to thank Advanstar together with NCC, Manchester (UK), and the UK CSVC for permission to draw on that material. Thanks are also due to HMSO (Crown copyright, for permission to use Figure 13.5), to Logica Industry Ltd and the Pharmaceutical Industry Computer Systems Validation Forum for permission to reproduce Figures 13.6 and 13.7, from the draft guideline "Validation of Automated Systems in Pharmaceutical Manufacturing". (24)

I should like to express my sincere thanks to the other authors contributing to this book for constructive peer reviews, to the many professionals in the industry who have stimulated thought and given advice to me in this rapidly advancing subject area, and to the management of the Medicines Control Agency in London for allowing me to contribute my views to this publication.

Last, but not least, my thanks are due to Amy Davis and Jane Steinmann for great patience in dealing with the "iterative" manuscript series process at Interpharm Press.

REFERENCES

1. Advanstar Communications, *Conference Proceedings:* The First European Pharmaceutical Technology Conference, 13–14 September 1993, Dusseldorf: Dean, D. M. Young, T. Comstock, pp. 394–400; Diederich, A., pp. 328–337; Korblein, G., pp. 121–129; Takashima, T., pp. 162–179; Warner, M., pp. 420–430 (Advanstar Communications, Advanstar House, Park West, Sealand Road, Chester, CH1 4RN, UK).

2. Trill, Tony, An Inspector's Thoughts on Pharmaceutical Production (Process Control). *Manufacturing Chemist* 61 (6): 31–35, June 1990.

3. Monger P, Packaging Security in the Pharmaceutical Industry: An MCA Inspector's Viewpoint. *Pharm. Technol. Int.* 5 (5): 50–53, May 1993.

4. Advanstar, 1993.

5. Ibid.

6. Rules and Guidance for Pharmaceutical Manufacturers (1993) incorporating the EC Guide to GMP, EC Directives on GMP, the Code of Practice for Qualified Persons, and Standard Provisions for Manufacturer's Licences. Published by HMSO for MCA. £11.50 net. ISBN 0-11-321633-5. (HMSO Publications Centre: PO Box 276, London, SW8 5DT, UK; Fax orders +44 71 873 8200).

7. Annex 11 to Volume IV of the Rules Governing Medicinal Products in the European Community (incorporated in Rules and Guidance for Pharmaceutical Manufacturers above), *Computerized Systems,* (from Working Paper draft 111/8263/89-EN of September 1989).

8. PRINCE (PRojects IN Controlled Environments) Structured Methodology for Project Management, National Computing Centre (NCC), Manchester M1 7ED, England, 1988.

9. SSADM (Structured System And Design Methodology) (CCTA/NCC) National Computing Centre (NCC), Manchester M1 7ED, England.

10. NAMAS Directory of Accredited Laboratories (electrical, electronic, IT, & telecommunications products testing), NAMAS Executive, National Physical Laboratory, Teddington, Middlesex TW11 0LW, UK.

11. Trill, A. J., Computerized Systems and GMP—A UK Perspective: Part I: Background, Standards, and Methods. *Pharm. Technol. Int.* 5 (2): 12–26, Feb.1993; Part II: Inspection Findings. *Pharm. Technol. Int.* 5 (3): 49–63, March 1993; Part III: Best Practices and Topical Issues. *Pharm. Technol. Int.* 5 (5): 17–30, May 1993.

12. NCC Publications, *The STARTS Purchaser's Handbook— Software Tools for Large Real Time Systems* (1986). *The STARTS Guide* (1987), ISBN 0-85012-619-3. *The IT STARTS Developer's Guide* (1988) ISBN 0-85012-733-5. NCC Publications, The National Computing Centre, Oxford Road, Manchester M1 7ED, England.

13. PMA/CSVC.

14. *TickIT (EN29001) Scheme for Software Sector Quality Certification*, DTI London 1989/1990 and related quality assessment guides and schedules (3302 series linking with BS 5750 (1 & 2) and EN29001 and 29002). The TickIT Guide (ISBN 0-9519309-0-7) Issue 2, price £25.00, incorporates ISO 9000-3 and is available from the DISC Office, together with a newsletter, case studies, and listings of TickIT certified firms. (DISC TickIT Office, 2 Park Street, London W1A 2BS (Tel:+44(0)71 602 8536; Fax:+44(0)71 602 8912).

15. **Quality System Standards—Guidelines**

    • ISO 9000: Quality Management and Quality Assurance Standards

    • ISO 9000-1: Guide for selection and use of applicable standards (1987)

- ISO 9000-2: Guide to the application of ISO 9001/2/3 (to replace BS 5750 Part 4: 1990)

- ISO 9000-3: Guidelines for the application of ISO 9001 to the development, supply, and maintenance of software (1991)

- ISO 9004: Quality Management and Quality Assurance Standards (1987)

  —Part 1: Guide to quality management and quality system elements (to be revised) (1987)

  —Part 2: Guidelines for services (1991)

  —Part 3: Guidelines for processed material

  —Part 4: Guidelines for managing quality improvement (in preparation—expected 1994/1995)

  —Part 5: Guidelines for Quality Plans

  —Part 6: Guidelines for Configuration Management (draft due 1993/1994)

- ISO 8402: Quality vocabulary

- ISO 2382: Data processing vocabulary

- BS 5515: Documentation of Computer-Based Systems

- BS 5887: Testing of Computer-Based Systems

- BS 6238: Performance Monitoring of Computer-Based Systems

ANSI/IEEE STANDARDS

- ANSI/IEEE 729: Standard Glossary of Software Engineering Terminology (1983)

- ANSI/IEEE 730: Software Quality Assurance Plans (1984)

- ANSI/IEEE 828: Software Configuration Management Plans (1983)

- ANSI/IEEE 829: Software Test Documentation (1983)

- ANSI/IEEE 830: Software Requirements Specifications (1984)

- ANSI/IEEE 983: Software QA Planning (1986)
- IEEE 990: Ada as a Program Design Language (1986)
- ANSI/IEEE 1002: Taxonomy for Software Engineering Standards (1987)
- ANSI/IEEE 1008: Software Unit Testing (1987)
- ANSI/IEEE 1012: Software Verification and Validation Plans (1986)
- IEEE 1016: Software Design Descriptions (1987)

(Published by The Institute of Electrical and Electronic Engineers, 345 E. 47th Street, New York, NY 10017, USA.)

Other Standards

- ISO DIS 10012: Quality Assurance Requirements for Measurement Equipment
- BS 7649: British Standard Guide to the design and preparation of documentation for users of application software (1993)
- BS 7850: Total Quality Management

  —Part 1: Guide to Management Principles (1992)

  —Part 2: Guide to Quality Improvement Methods (1992)
- DIN 66 285: Information Processing Application Software—Quality requirements and testing
- INTDEF-STAN 00-55: Procurement of Safety Critical Software in Defense Equipment (1991)
- INTDEF-STAN 00-56: Hazard Analysis and Safety Classification of Computer and Programmable System Elements (1991)

16. EOQC, *Seminar Proceedings:* 1 Seminaire E.O.Q.C. Sur la Qualité des Logiciels. (First European Seminar on Software Quality), Brussels, 25–27 April 1988.

17. Logica, *Quality Management Standards for Software.* A report prepared by Logica for the UK Department of Trade and Industry (Ref: 621.6693), April 1988.

18. Price-Waterhouse, *Software Quality Standards: The Costs and Benefits*. A review for the UK Department of Trade and Industry, April 1988.

19. TickIT, 1990.

20. Management Forum Seminars, *Standards for Computerized Systems:* Banks, A. G., G. Cassford, A. J. Margetts, A. J. Trill (Management Forum Ltd., 48 Woodbridge Road, Guildford, Surrey GU1 4RJ, UK).

21. Trill, 1993.

22. PICSVF, *Good Automated Manufacturing Practice in the Pharmaceutical Industry (GAMP)*, Conference and launch of Draft Guidelines. "Validation of Automated Systems in Pharmaceutical Manufacturing," 1 March 1994, Queen Elizabeth II Conference Centre, London. (Management Forum Ltd). NB: Guidelines to be published by Logica Industry Ltd. Units A & E, Business Park No. 4, Randalls Research Park, Randalls Way, Leatherhead, Surrey KT 22 7TW, UK (draft available).

23. Trill, 1993.

24. PICSVF, 1994.

Appendix *A*
Acronyms

Kenneth G. Chapman

LEGEND
1	= Regulatory Agency	6	= Regulations
2	= GMP-related	7	= Tech./Prof./Trade Assoc
3	= GLP-related	8	= Software-related
4	= GCP-related	9	= New Product related
5	= Standards-related	10	= General

ACRONYM	MEANING	
ADR	Adverse Drug Reaction	4
AE	Adverse Event	4
ANDA	Abbreviated New Drug Application	2
ANSI	American National Standard Institute	5
APEC	Asia-Pacific Economic Cooperation	10
ASEAN	Association of South Eastern Asian Nations	10
ASCII	American Standard Code for Information Interchange	5
BGA	Bundesgesundheitsamtes (German)	1
BPC	Bulk Pharmaceutical Chemical	10
CANDA	Computer Assisted New Drug Application	9
CAD	Computer Assisted Design	8
CAM	Computer Assisted Manufacturing	8
CASE	Computer Assisted Software Engineering	8
CBER	Center for Biologics Evaluation & Research (US FDA)	1

CDER	Center for Drug Evaluation & Research (US FDA)	1
CEC	Commission of the European Communities	1
CFR	Code of Federal Regulations (US)	6
CGMPs	Current GMPs (US)	6
CFR	Code of Federal Regulations (US)	6
CIM	Computer Integrated Manufacturing	2
COTS	Commercial Off-The-Shelf (US)	8
CPMP	Committee for Proprietary Medicinal Products (EC)	1
CRF	Case Report Form	4
CSVC	Computer System Validation Committee (of PMA, US)	7
DAMOS	Drug Application Methodology with Optical Storage	8
DIA	Drug Information Association (US)	7
DMF	Drug Master File (FDA)	6
EBR	Electronic Batch Record	2
EC	Former European Community, now European Union	10
EC	European Commission of EC/EU	10
EDI	Electronic Data Interchange	10
EFPIA	European Federation of Pharmaceutical Industry Association	7
eID	Electronic Identification	8
EP	European Pharmacopoeia	5
EPA	Environmental Protection Agency (US)	1
EU	European Union (former EC)	10
FDA	Food & Drug Administration (US)	1
FOI	Freedom of Information (FDA)	6
GALP	Good Automated Laboratory Practices (US EPA)	5
GATT	General Agreement on Tariffs & Trade	10
GCP	Good Clinical Practices	4
GDEA	Generic Drug Enforcement Act of 1992 (FDA)	6
GLP	Good Laboratory Practices [laboratory]	10
GLP	Good Laboratory Practices [Preclinical]	3
GMP	Good Manufacturing Practices	2
GSEP	Good Software Engineering Practices	8
HIMA	Health Industries Manufacturers Association	7
IEEE	Institute of Electrical & Electronics Engineers	5
IES	Institute of Environmental Sciences	7
IIR	Institute for International Research (US)	7
IND	Investigational New Drug Application (US)	9
IQ	Installation Qualification	10
IS	Information Services	7

ISO	International Standards Organization	5
ISPE	International Society for Pharmaceutical Engineering	7
IT	Information Technology	7
JP	Japanese Pharmacopoeia	5
JPMA	Japanese Pharmaceutical Manufacturers Association	7
LIMS	Laboratory Information Management System	2
MMI	Man/Machine Interface	10
MCA	Medicines Control Agency (UK)	1
MRP	Manufacturing Resource Planning	2
MRP	Materials Requirement Planning	2
NAFTA	North American Free Trade Agreement	10
NCSL	National Conference of Standards Laboratories (US)	5
NDA	New Drug Application (US)	9
NDMA	Nonprescription Drug Manufacturers Association (US)	7
NIST	National Institute of Standards & Technology (US)	5
OCR	Optical Character Recognition	8
OGD	Office of Generic Drugs (FDA)	1
OOS	Out Of Specifications	10
OQ	Operational Qualification	10
PDA	Parenteral Drug Assoc. (US)	7
PDMA	Prescription Drug Manufacturing Act (FDA)	6
PQ	Performance Qualification	10
PIC	Pharmaceutical Inspection Commission	2
PMA	Pharmaceutical Manufacturers' Assoc. (US)	7
QA	Quality Assurance	10
QC	Quality Control	10
RAPS	Regulatory Affairs Professional Society (US)	7
RFP	Request for Proposal (or Purchase)	7
RIBS	References for Investigative Branches (FDA)	2
ROI	Return-on-Investment	10
SCADA	Supervisory Control Data Acquisition	10
SDLC	System Development Life Cycle	10
SFSTP	Societe Francaise Des Sciences et Techniques Pharmaceutiques (Fr.)	7
SGML	Standard Generalised Markup Language	5
SQA	Software Quality Assurance	8
SQAP	Software Quality Assurance Plan	8
TGA	Therapeutic Goods Administration (Australia)	1
USP	US Pharmacopoeia	5
WHO	World Health Organization	10

Appendix *B*
Glossary

Kenneth G. Chapman

Author's Note: The following is a selection of terms deemed likely to be useful to the readers. Associated definitions reflect what this author believes to be the most applicable contemporary interpretations of terminology originally published by various authorities, ranging from Dr. J. M. Juran to IEEE/ANSI and including PMA, PDA, and many other authors.

Acceptance Criteria (Software):   The criteria a software product must meet to successfully complete a test phase or to achieve delivery requirements.

Action Levels: Levels of ranges distinct from product specifications that, when deviated from, signal a drift from normal operating conditions and that require action.

Alert Levels: Levels or ranges that, when deviated from, signal a potential drift from normal operating conditions but that do not necessarily require action.

Application-Specific Software: Software written to a specified user requirement for the purpose of performing unique designated task(s); includes Customized Configurable.

Boundary Value: A data value that corresponds to a minimum or maximum input, internal, or output value specified for a system or component.

Branch Testing: Execution of enough tests to assure that every Branch Alternative has been exercised at least once.

Bug: A manifestation of an error in software (a fault).

Calibration: Demonstration that a particular measuring device produces results within specified limits by comparison with those produced by a reference standard device over an appropriate range of measurements. This process results in correction that may be applied to optimize accuracy.

Canned Configurable Software: Commercial, off-the-shelf software that can be configured to specific user applications by "filling in the blanks," without altering the basic program.

Change Control: A formal system by which qualified representatives of appropriate disciplines review proposed or actual changes that might affect a validated status. The intent is to determine the need for action that would ensure and document that the system is maintained in a validated state.

Common Sense: Thought process that emphasizes use of ordinary logic and deductive reasoning.

Computer System: A group of hardware components and associated software designed and assembled to perform a specific function or group of functions. (CSVC)

Computerized System: Computer system plus any subsystem(s) it controls.

Computer-Related System: Computerized system plus its Operating Environment.

Concurrent Process Validation: Establishing documented evidence that a process does what it purports to do based on information generated during actual implementation of the process.

Critical Process Parameter: A process-related variable that, when out-of-control, can potentially cause an adverse effect on fitness-for-use of an end product.

Custom Configurable Software: Canned Configurable software that has been modified to meet specific needs of an end user with the addition of new system functionality by means of additional programming (thereby converting it to Application Software).

Debugging: The process of locating, analyzing, and correcting suspected faults.

Documentation: Any written or pictorial information describing, defining, specifying, and/or reporting of certifying activities, requirements, procedures, or results.

Edge-of-Failure: A control parameter value that, if exceeded, means adverse effect on state of control and/or fitness for use of the product.

Electronic Verification: An input command that enables a designated user, or the computerized system itself, to electronically signify verification or endorsement of a specific step, transaction, or data entry. The source of the electronic verification may be made visible or invisible to users of the data.

Ergonomics: The study of human interaction with machines.

Executive Program: A computer program, usually part of the operating system, that controls the execution of other computer programs and regulates the flow of work in a data processing system.

Functional Requirements: Requirements that specify functions a system or system component must be capable of performing.

Functional Testing: Also known as black box testing, since source code is not needed. Involves inputting normal and abnormal test cases; then evaluating the outputs against those expected. Can apply to computer software or to a total system (*See also* Performance Qualification).

High-Level Language: A computer programming language that approaches human-spoken languages (e.g., English, French, German) in its syntax. Usually easier to learn than a low-level language, such as assembly language.

Installation Qualification (IQ):   Documented verification that all key aspects of the installation adhere to approved design intentions according to system specifications and that manufacturers' recommendations are suitably considered.

Life Cycle Concept (Validation):   An approach to validating a computer-related system that begins with identification of the user's requirements, continues though design, integration, qualification, acceptance and maintenance, and ends only when commercial use of the system is discontinued.

Machine Code: A representation of instructions and data that is directly executable by a computer (machine language).

Modularity (Software):   The extent to which software is composed of discrete components such that a change to one component has minimal impact on other components.

Object Code: The Machine-code program produced by a compiler or assembler.

Operating Environment: Those activities interfacing directly or indirectly with the system of concern, control of which can affect the system's validated state.

Operating System: A set of programs provided with a computer that functions as the interface between the hardware and the application programs.

Operating System Software: Software that controls the execution of programs.

Operational Qualification (OQ):   Documented verification that each unit or subsystem operates as intended throughout its anticipated operating range.

Performance Qualification (PQ):   Documented verification that the integrated system performs as intended in its normal operating environment.

Peripheral: A device other than the computer itself used in computer processing. Disk drives, tape drives, CRTs, and printers are peripheral devices.

Policy: A directive usually specifying what is to be accomplished.

Procedure: A directive usually specifying how certain activities are to be accomplished.

Prospective Validation: Establishing documented evidence that a system does what it purports to do based on a validation plan.

Protocol (Qualification Protocol):   A prospective experimental plan that when executed is intended to produce documented evidence that a system or subsystem has been properly qualified.

Proven Acceptable Ranges (PAR):   All values of a given control parameter that fall between established high and low boundary conditions.

Quality Assurance (QA):   The activity of providing the evidence needed to establish confidence that the quality function is being performed adequately.

Quality Control (QC): The regulatory process through which industry measures actual quality performance, compares it with standards, and acts on the difference.

Quality Function: The entire collection of activities from which industry achieves fitness for use, no matter where these activities are performed.

Requalification: Repetition of a qualification exercise or a portion thereof.

Retroactive Process Validation: Establishing documented evidence that a system does what it purports to do after the system is used for commercial purposes.

Retrospective Validation: Establishing documented evidence that a system does what it purports to do based on review and analysis of historic information.

Revalidation: Repetition of the validation process or a specific portion of it.

Robustness: The degree to which a system or subsystem can continue to function reliably and reproducibly under sustained operation and actual environmental conditions.

Security: The protection of computer hardware and software from accidental or malicious access, use, modification, destruction, or disclosure. Security also pertains to personnel, data, communications, and the physical protection of computer installations.

Software: (1) A collection of programs, routines, and subroutines that controls the operation of a computer or a computerized system; (2) A set of programs, procedures, rules, and associated documentation concerned with the operation of a computer system (e.g., compilers, library routines, and manuals); (3) A program package containing instructions for the computer hardware.

Software Life Cycle: The period of time that starts when a software product is conceived and ends when the product is no longer available for use. The software life cycle typically includes a requirements phase, design phase, implementation phase, test phase, installation and checkout phase, and operation and maintenance phase.

Source Code: (1) An original computer program expressed in human-readable form (programming language), which must be translated into machine-readable form before it can be executed by the computer; (2) A program written in a computer language to be compiled or assembled into object code.

Statement Testing: Execution of all statements at least once; also known as node coverage.

State-of-Control: A condition in which all operating variables that can affect performance remain within such ranges that the system of process performs consistently and as intended.

Stress Testing: Testing conducted to evaluate a system or component at or beyond the limits of its specified requirements.

Structural Integrity: The degree to which source code adheres to software development procedures and prespecified standards.

Structural Testing: Examining the internal structure of the source code. Includes low-level and high-level code review, path analysis, auditing of programming procedures and standards actually used, inspection for extraneous "dead code," boundary analysis, and other techniques. Requires specific computer science and programming expertise.

Structural Verification: Detailed examination of the functional logic of source code to verify that it conforms to specified software requirements, and inspection of the program for adherence to software development procedures.

System Software: Software designed to facilitate the operation and maintenance of a computer system and its associated programs, such as operating systems, assemblers, utilities, and executive programs. System software is generally independent of the specific application.

System Specifications: (1) Software designed for a specific computer system or family of computer systems to facilitate the operation and maintenance of the computer system and associated programs (e.g., operating systems, compilers, utilities); (2) Document that describes how a system will meet its functional requirements.

Top-Down Design: An organization of design where plans are made for modules arranged in a pyramid, starting at the top-most module, which is the most generalized concept of the control system.

Uninterruptible Power Supply (UPS):   A power supply having back-up battery storage. A UPS is used to ensure operation of critical computer equipment during power failures.

Validation: Establishing documented evidence that provides a high degree of assurance that a specific system will consistently produce a product meeting its predetermined specifications and quality attributes.

Validation Project Plan ("Master Plan"): A document that identifies all systems and subsystems involved in a specific validation effort and the approach by which they will be qualified and the total system validated; includes identification of responsibilities and expectations.

Worst Case: (1) A set of conditions encompassing upper and lower processing limits and circumstances, including those within standard operation procedures, which pose the greatest chance of process or product failure when compared to ideal conditions. Such conditions do not necessarily induce product or process failure; (2) The highest or lowest boundary value of a given control parameter actually established in a validation qualification exercise.

Appendix C
Drumbeat™ Analysis (1)

Kenneth G. Chapman

The following table illustrates a useful system for analyzing requirements that are based on various regulations or guidelines. The DRUM-BEAT system (2) was developed in 1977 by this author and used to survey all of Pfizer's GMP-related policies and procedures against new regulatory requirements existing or emerging at the time. DRUMBEAT was later adapted to other uses, such as appraising document quality and ensuring document availability.

To analyze requirements, a list of concepts is prepared, based on common sense, experience, and surveys of relevant regulations and guidelines. Each concept should represent a single thought or activity, overlapping other concepts to the least possible extent. Most of the concepts in Appendices C, D, and E are developed from the Computer System Validation Life Cycle.

As can be seen in this appendix, European Commission GMPs (3) and Australian GMPs (4) match each other fairly closely; Appendices D and E provide the exact wording of each document for comparison purposes. U.S. GMPs (5) provide minimal specifications, in keeping with FDA's tradition of stating in its GMPs only what is to be accomplished, and not how to accomplish it. Many DRUMBEAT concepts can be related to portions of ISO-9000-3 (6), but close examination of the ISO-9000 wording reveals that it generally lacks the kind of technological substance found in most other references (i.e., ISO-9000 standards provide useful discipline in calling for procedures to be available, but offer little advice concerning what those procedures should contain). The 1986 PMA Concept Paper (7) is not indexed in a manner that facilitates such analysis, a point to be kept in mind when developing new guidelines.

Besides being useful for reconciling existing documents against requirements, tables of this kind can also provide helpful reminders when developing a Project Validation Plan, teaching a course, or developing new policies, procedures, and guidelines.

Drumbeat™	EC GMP Annex 11	Aus. GMPs	US GMPs	PDA Mono- graph	PMA Con- cept Paper	ISO- 9000-3
Reference	8	9	10	11	12	13
2.05 *Computer-Related System Validation* Validating systems in which one or more microprocessors are utilized as part of a control or data pro- cessing function.						
2.05.01 *System Definition* Providing clear de- scriptions of the phys- ical system and of its intended functions.	3 18	905		3.1, 4.2.1, 4.4	√	5.3.1
2.05.02 *Software Quality Assurance Plan (SQAP)* Describing the way software is developed, including conventions and standards to be used, annotation requirements, quality assurance measures, change control and archival practices. SQAP objective is to establish structural quality of software.	4	904		4.3.2, 4.5.2, 4.5.3	√	4.2.3, 5.6.3a

Drumbeat™	EC GMP Annex 11	Aus. GMPs	US GMPs	PDA Mono-graph	PMA Con-cept Paper	ISO-9000-3
2.05.03 *Installation Qualification* Providing documented verification that all key aspects of hardware installation adhere to appropriate codes and approved design intentions and supplier recommendations have been suitably considered.				4.6	√	5.9.3 e,f
2.05.04 *Operational Qualification* Providing documented verification that each subsystem performs as intended throughout its representative or anticipated operating ranges.				4.6	√	
2.05.05 *Functional Test Protocol* Providing an experimental plan that is intended, when executed, to produce documented evidence that the system functions as intended in its operating environment and under all normal and outer-boundary conditions to be realistically expected.	6 (par-allel)	906		4.6	√	5.7.1 5.7.2

Drumbeat™	EC GMP Annex 11	Aus. GMPs	US GMPs	PDA Mono-graph	PMA Con-cept Paper	ISO-9000-3
2.05.06 *Protocol Execution* Executing the functional test protocol, reviewing results and approving documented conclusions.	6	906		4.6.3	√	5.7.3
2.05.07 *Change Control, Revalidation* Providing a monitoring system by which appropriate formal reviews and approvals are made of proposed or actual changes, of the kind that might affect a system's validated status; includes determining need for corrective revalidation action and then effecting and documenting that action.	10	907		4.7.1	√	6.1.1 6.1.3
2.05.08 *Ongoing Q.A. Evaluation* Providing system audits and periodic reviews of all changes to seek potential cumulative effects that might warrant revalidation.	12	917		4.7, 4.7.7, 4.7.8	√	

Drumbeat™	EC GMP Annex 11	Aus. GMPs	US GMPs	PDA Mono-graph	PMA Con-cept Paper	ISO-9000-3
2.05.09 *Security - Human Involvement* Providing measures to permit only autho-rized access to hard-ware and software components of com-puter systems, to prevent unintended and unauthorized changes.	7 9	911		4.7.3	√	
2.05.10 *Security - Environment* Protecting the system against damage, al-teration or loss of data from such envi-ronmental factors as vibration, electro-mechanical noise and excessive humidity or temperature condi-tions.	2 12	916			√	
2.05.11 *Data Input Assurance* Assuring correctness of system input data, either by human intervention, such as dual witnessing, or through design of the computerized system and its operating environment.	5 8	910	.68 b			

Drumbeat™	EC GMP Annex 11	Aus. GMPs	US GMPs	PDA Mono-graph	PMA Con-cept Paper	ISO-9000-3
2.05.12 *Contingency and Recovery* Identifying circumstances, such as power loss and catastrophic events, that could jeopardize the system database, software or hardware, and providing contingency and recovery measures designed to preserve integrity of the system and to protect fitness-for-use of any product involved.	13 14 15	913		4.7.4	√	
2.05.13 *Data Inspection Access* Providing capability to generate electronic or paper copies of contained data for inspection purposes.	11	914				
2.05.14 *Outside Computer Service* Providing a formal agreement to designate responsibilities whenever an outside agency provides computer services.	17					

Drumbeat™	EC GMP Annex 11	Aus. GMPs	US GMPs	PDA Mono-graph	PMA Con-cept Paper	ISO-9000-3
2.05.16 *Error Handling* Providing a SOP to record and analyze errors and to enable corrective actions.	16					6.4.1
2.05.17 *Limiting Use* Restricting computer-ized systems to des-ignated use and al-lowing only systems meeting SQA re-quirements to be used.	18				√	

REFERENCES

1. DRUMBEAT™ copyright is assigned to Pfizer Inc.

2. K. G. Chapman, "A Procedural Approach to Quality Assurance," *Pharm. Tech. Conference 1982*, 45–60, (September 1982).

3. Commission of the European Communities, "Computerized Systems," *Annex 11 to Good Manufacturing Practice for Medicinal Products in the European Community*, (January, 1992).

4. Therapeutic Goods Administration, "Use of Computers," *Australian Code of GMP for Therapeutic Goods—Medicinal Products—Part 1 Section 9*, (January, 1993).

5. FDA, "Human and Veterinary Drugs, Current Good Manufacturing Practice in Manufacture, Processing, Packing or Holding," *Federal Register*, 43, No. 190, 45014–45089, (29 September 1978).

6. *International Standard ISO 9000-3*, "Quality Management and Quality Assurance Standards—Part 3: Guidelines for the Application of ISO 9001 to the Development, Supply and Maintenance of Software," International Organization for Standardization, Geneva, 1st ed., 1–15, (1991-06-01).

7. PMA's Computer Systems Validation Committee, "Validation Concepts for Computer Systems Used in the Manufacture of Drug Products," *Pharm. Technol.* 10 (5), 24–34 (1986).

8. Commission of the European Communities, 1992.

9. Therapeutic Goods Administration, "Use of Computers," *Australian Code of GMP for Therapeutic Goods—Medicinal Products—*Part 1 Section 9, (January, 1993).

10. FDA, 29 September 1978.

11. Parenteral Drug Association (PDA), "Validation of Computer-Related Systems," pre-publication monograph manuscript (October, 1993).

12. PMA, 1986.

13. *International Standard ISO 9000-3* (Refers only to software).

Appendix **D**

European Commission GMP Annex 11 Analysis

Kenneth G. Chapman

There follows a list of the 19 concepts that constitute Annex 11 of the Guide to Good Manufacturing Practice for Medicinal Products from Volume IV of the *Rules Governing Medicinal Products in the European Community* (now, European Union). These concepts closely resemble similar concepts in the DRUMBEAT™ system and in the Australian GMPs. Actual relationships are identified in the table that follows, and also in Appendices C and E.

Annex 11, *Computerized Systems*, begins with the following Principle:

> The introduction of computerized systems into systems of manufacturing, including storage, distribution, and quality control does not alter the need to observe the relevant principles given elsewhere in the Guide. Where a computerized system replaces a manual operation, there should be no resultant decrease in product quality or quality assurance. Consideration should be given to the risk of losing aspects of the previous system which could result from reducing the involvement of operators.

EC GMP Annex 11	Drumbeat™	Aus GMPs
PERSONNEL		
1. It is essential that there is the closest cooperation between key personnel and those involved with computer systems. Persons in responsible positions should have the appropriate training for the management and use of systems within their field of responsibility which utilizes computers. This should include ensuring that appropriate expertise is available and use to provide advice on aspects of design, validation, installation and operation of computerized system.		
SYSTEM		
2. Attention should be paid to the siting of equipment in suitable conditions where extraneous factors cannot interfere with the system.	2.05.10	916
3. A detailed description of the system should be produced (including diagrams as appropriate) and kept up to date. It should describe the principles. Objectives, security measures and scope of the system and the main features of the way in which the computer is used and how it interacts with other systems and procedures.	2.05.01	905
4. The software is a critical component of a computerized system. The user of such software should take all necessary steps to insure that it has been produced in accordance with a system of Quality Assurance.	2.05.02	904

EC GMP Annex 11	Drumbeat™	Aus GMPs
5. The system should include, where appropriate, built-in checks of the correct entry and processing of data.	2.05.11	910
6. Before a system using a computer is brought into use. It should be tested and confirmed as being capable of achieving the desired results. If a manual system is being replaced, it is advisable to run the two in parallel for a time, as part of this testing and validation.	2.05.05 2.05.06	906 (Parallel)
7. Data should only be entered or amended by persons authorized to do so. Suitable methods of deterring unauthorized entry of data include the use of keys, pass cards, personal codes and restricted access to com-puter terminals.	2.05.09	911
8. When critical data are being entered manually (for example the weight and batch number of an ingredient during dispensing), there should be and independent check on the accu-racy of the record which is made. The system should also record the identity of the operator(s) involved.	2.05.11 5.11	910
9. There should be a defined procedure for the issue, cancellation and alter-ation of authorization to amend data. Including the changing of personal codes. Authority to alter entered data should be restricted to nominated persons. Any alteration to an entry of critical data should be authorized and recorded with the reason for the change.	2.05.09	91

EC GMP Annex 11	Drumbeat™	Aus GMPs
10. Alterations to a system or to a computer programme should only be made in accordance with a defined procedure which should include provision for checking, approving and implementing the change. Such an alteration should only be implemented with the agreement of the person responsible for the part of the system concerned, and the alteration should be recorded.	2.05.07	907
11. It must be possible to obtain meaningful printed copies of electronically stored data which relates to a process which would normally be required for quality auditing purpose.	2.05.13*	914
12. Data should be secured against wilful or accidental damage by personnel or by physical or electronic means and in accordance with item 4.9 of the guide. Stored data should be checked for accessibility, durability and accuracy. If changes are proposed to the computer equipment or its programmes, the above checks should be performed at a frequency appropriate to the storage medium being used.	2.05.10 2.05.08	916 917
13. Data should be protected by backing-up at regular intervals. Back-up data should be stored at a separate and secure location.	2.05.12	913
14. There should be available adequate alternative arrangements for systems which need to be operated in the event of a breakdown. The time required to bring the alternative arrangements into use should be related to the possible urgency of the need to use them. For example, information required to effect a recall must be available at short notice.	2.05.12	913

EC GMP Annex 11	Drumbeat™	Aus GMPs
15. The procedures to be followed if the system fails or breaks down should be defined and validated at regular intervals. Any failures and remedial action taken should be recorded.	2.05.12	913
16. A procedure should be established to record and analyze errors and to enable corrective action to be taken.	2.05.16	
17. When outside agencies are used to provide a computer service, there should be a formal agreement including a clear statement of the responsibilities of that outside agency (see Chapter 7).	2.05.14	
18. Computerized systems should be restricted to their designed use. Only these systems conforming with item 4 should be used. Reasonable precautions should be taken to protect the system against outside influences.	2.05.17	
19. When the release of batches for sale or supply is ensured by a computerized system, it should recognize that only a Qualified Person can release the batches and it should clearly identify the person releasing the batches.	6.16	

Appendix *E*

Australian Code of GMP Analysis

Kenneth G. Chapman

The following table lists 18 concepts that constitute Section 9, *Use of Computers*, of the Australian Code of GMP for Therapeutic Goods—Medicinal Products Part 1. These concepts closely resemble similar concepts in the DRUMBEAT™ system and in the EC GMPs Annex 11. Actual relationships are identified in the table that follows, and also in Appendices C and D.

The key point to note is the global harmonization occurring with regard to validation of computer-related systems.

Australian Code of GMP	Drumbeat™	EC GMPs Annex 11
900. Where a computer is used in connection with any procedure or process associated with the production of therapeutic goods, the computer system employed should meet the requirements of this code for those manual functions which it replaces.		
901. The responsibilities of the key persons in manufacturing and quality departments are not changed by the use of computers.		
902. Persons with appropriate expertise should be responsible for the design, introduction and regular review of a computer system.		
903. The development, implementation and operation of a computer system should be carefully documented at all stages and each step proven to achieve its written objective under challenging test conditions.		
904. Software development should follow the principles of Australian Standard AS 3563: Software Quality Management System. A logic flow diagram of a schematic for software should be prepared for critical evaluation against system design/requirements/criteria.	2.05.02	4
905. A control document should be prepared specifying the objectives of a proposed computer system, the data to be entered and stored, the flow of data, the information to be produced, the limits of any variables and the operating program(s) and test programs, together with examples of each document produced by the program, instructions for testing, operating and maintaining the system and the names of the person or persons responsible for its development and operation.	2.05.01	3 18

Australian Code of GMP	Drumbeat™	EC GMPs Annex 11
906. When a computer system is in process of replacing a manual operation, the two systems should be operated in parallel until it has been shown that the computer system is operating correctly. Records of the parallel operation and the defects found and resolved should be added to the history document in the following Clause.	2.05.05 2.05.06	6 (parallel)
907. Any change to an existing computer system should be made in accordance with a defined change control procedure which should document the details of each change made, its purpose and its date of effect and should provide for a check to confirm that the change has been applied correctly.	2.05.07	10
908. Where development has progressed to a point where the system cannot readily be assessed by reading the control and development documents together, a new control document incorporating all amendments should be prepared and the original retained.		
909. Data collected directly from manufacturing or monitoring equipment should be checked by verifying circuits of software to confirm that it has been accurately and reliably transferred.		
910. The entry of critical data into a computer by an authorized person (e.g., entering a master processing formula) should require independent verification and release for use by a second authorized person.	2.05.11	5 8

Australian Code of GMP	Drumbeat™	EC GMPs Annex 11
911. A hierarchy of permitted access to enter, amend, read, or print out data should be established according to user need. Suitable methods of preventing unauthorized entry should be available, such as pass cards or personal user-identity codes. A list of forbidden codes, e.g., names, birthdays, should be issued and a procedure for regular change of codes should be established.	2.05.09	7 9
912. The computer system should create a complete record ("audit trail") of all entries and amendments to the data base.		
913. The recovery procedure to be followed in the event of a system breakdown should be defined in writing. This procedure should be designed to return the system to a previous state. A check should be made periodically that all programs and data necessary to restore the system will be available in case of breakdown. Any such breakdown and the recovery action taken should be recorded.	2.05.12	13 14 15
914. The computer system should be able to provide printed copies of relevant data and information stored within it. Hard copies of master documents should be signed, dated and filed in accordance with Section 5.	2.05.13	11
915. Printed matter produced by computer peripherals should be clearly legible and, in the case of printing onto forms, should be properly registered onto the forms.		

Australian Code of GMP	Drumbeat™	EC GMPs Annex 11
916. Storage of live and master data should be in accordance with Clauses 516 and 513 respectively.	2.05.10	2 12
917. Records should be available for the following aspects of a computer system validation: • Protocol for validation • General description of the system, the components and the operating characteristics. • Diagrams of hardware layout/interaction • List of programs with brief description of each. • System logic diagrams or other schematic form for software packages • Current configuration for hardware and software • Review of historical logs of hardware and software for development, start-up and normal run periods • Records of evaluation data to demonstrate system does as intended (verification stage and ongoing monitoring) • Range of limits for operation variables • Details of formal change control procedure • Records of operator training • Details of access security levels/controls • Procedure for ongoing evaluation	2.05.08	12

Appendix *F*
Recommended Reading

Anthony J. Trill

1. FDA, Guide to Inspection of Computerized Systems in Drug Processing (*The Blue Book*), Food and Drug Administration, Center for Drug Evaluation and Research, Rockville, MD, 1983.

2. *The Orange Guide*, The Guide to Good Pharmaceutical Manufacturing Practice, 1983. Crown Copyright, DHSS, Chapter 16. ISBN 011 3208324, £3.95.

3. Bonnes Pratiques de Fabrication et de Production Pharmaceutiques, 1985. French Ministry of Health. Chapter 18. ISSN 0758-1998 (9OF).

4. Norbert R. Kuzel, Fundamentals of Computer System Validation and Documentation in the Pharmaceutical Industry. *Pharm. Technol.*, pp. 60–60, Sept. 1985.

5. PMA's Computer Systems Validation Committee, Validation Concepts for Computer Systems Used in the Manufacture of Drug Products. *Pharm. Technol.*, pp. 24–34, May 1986.

6. J. Agalloco, Validation of Existing Systems. *Pharm. Technol.*, pp. 38–42, January 1987.

7. FDA, *Software Development Activities, Reference Materials, and Training Aids for Investigators.* Food and Drug Administration, Associate Commissioner for Regulatory Affairs, Division of Field Investigations, Rockville, MD, April 1987.

8. FDA, *Compliance Policy Guides on Computerized Drug Processing:* 7132a.07: Input-Output Checking; 7132a.08: Identification of Persons—Batch Control Records; 7132a.11: CGMP Applicability to Hardware and Software; 7132a.12: Vendor Responsibility; 7132a.15: Source Code for Process Control Application Programs. April 1987. (This and other guides in the series, available from Food and Drug Administration, Freedom of Information Staff, [HFI-35], 5600 Fishers Lane, Rockville, MD 20857).

9. 21 *Code of Federal Regulations*, Parts 210–211 (Current Good Manufacturing Practice). U.S. FDA, Rockville, MD.

10. Norbert R. Kuzel, Quality Assurance Auditing of Computer Systems. *Pharm.Technol.*, pp. 34–42, February 1987.

11. K. G. Chapman, et al., Source Code Availability and Vendor-User Relationships. *Pharm. Technol.*, pp. 24–35, December 1987.

12. Y. S. Gudesblat, Software Validation in Pharmaceutical Manufacture. *Programmable Controls*, pp. 34–37, May/June, 1988.

13. A. Samuel Clark, Computer Systems Validation: An Investigator's View. *Pharm. Technol.*, pp. 60–66, January 1988.

14. E. Doubek and W. Polonius, Computer Systems Validation. *Drugs Made in Germany*, 31 (1): 23–38, 1988.

15. A. J. Trill, Approaches to the Validation of Computer Systems in Quality Assurance. *Proceedings of Symposium: Computer Applications in Pharmaceutical Quality Assurance*, 9 June 1988, The Institute of Quality Assurance, London, England.

16. E. M. Fry, FDA Regulation of Computer Systems in Drug Manufacturing. *Pharm. Engineering* 8 (5): 50, Sept/Oct 1988.

17. J. P. Jeater and A. J. Margetts, Validation of Computer Systems used for Process Control and Management Information. ICI Pharmaceuticals, Macclesfield, Cheshire, UK, *Proceedings of Interphex '88*, The National Exhibition Centre, Birmingham, England, November 1988.

18. R. D. McDowall, J. C. Pearce, and G. S. Murkitt, Laboratory Information Management Systems—Part I: Concepts and Part II: Implementation. SK & F Research, Welwyn, UK, in *Journal of Pharmaceutical & Biomedical Analysis* 6 (4): 339–359, 1988; and 6 (4): 361–381, 1988.

19. K. G. Chapman, Computer System Regulation: Seeking Common Ground. *Pharm. Technol.* 13 (6): 16, 18, June 1989.

20. Council Directive 91/356/EEC of 13 June 1991 laying down the principles and guidelines of good manufacturing practice for medicinal products for human use (O.J. No. L 193 of 17 July 1991).

21. Council Directive 91/412/EEC of 23 July 1991 laying down the principles and guidelines of good manufacturing practice for veterinary medicinal products (O.J. No. L 228 of 17 August 1991).

22. K. G. Chapman, FDA Regulation of Computerized Systems, Keele University Conference and K. G. Chapman, J. Agallaco, et al., Computer System Validation—Staying Current, etc. *Pharm. Technol.* (various) 1989–1990.

23. *Proceedings of Training Course and Conference:* Assessing Computerized Systems in the Pharmaceutical Industry. MCA Medicines Inspectorate, Keele University, April 1989.

24. R. Geschwandtner, Validation of Computer Assisted Production Processes in Pharmaceutical Manufacturing. *Die Pharmazeutische Industrie* 51 (8),: 911–913, August 1989.

25. The Rules Governing Medicinal Products in the European Community, Vols I to V, January 1989.

26. The Institute of Quality Assurance, *Quality Assessment Schedules for Suppliers of Starting Materials to the Pharmaceutical Industry.* (IQA, 10 Grosvenor Gardens, London SW1W 0DQ).

27. A. J. Trill, A Medicines Inspector's Views on Validation Requirements for Computerized Systems in the European Drug Processing Industry. *Pharma Technologie Journal* 11 (3): 86–98, 1990; also in *Proceedings of Concept Symposium: Validierung von Computersystemen in der Pharma-Industrie, October 1990, Frankfurt am Main, Germany.*

28. A. P. van Oyen, Integrated Computer Applications for Pharmaceutical Manufacturing. In *Sterile Pharmaceutical Manufacturing Applications for the 1990's*, Volume 1, pp. 25–42, edited by M. J. Groves, W. P. Olson, M. H. Anisfeld, Interpharm Press Inc., 1991 (ISBN: 0-935184-21-X).

29. R. F. Tetzlaff, GMP Documentation Requirements for Automated Systems: Part I. *Pharm. Technol.*, pp. 112–124, March 1992.

30. R. F. Tetzlaff, GMP Documentation Requirements for Automated Systems: Part II. *Pharm. Technol.*, pp. 60–72, April 1992.

31. R. F. Tetzlaff, GMP Documentation Requirements for Automated Systems: Part III, FDA Inspections of Computerized Laboratory Systems. *Pharm.Technol.*, pp. 70–83, May 1992.

32. K. G. Chapman, Worldwide Opportunities Through Validation. *STP Pharma Pratiques* 2 (5): 415–422, 1992 (XXIV session de formation SFSTP de Montpellier).

33. Quality Control Reports, *The Gold Sheet* 26 (8), August 1992, Electronic Identifications. (F-D-C Reports Inc., Chevy Chase, MD 20815-7278).

34. P. J. Motise, FDA Considerations on Electronic Identification and Signatures. *Pharm. Technol.* 16 (11): 29–35, 77, 1992; and *Pharm. Technol. Int.*, pp. 24–32, 55, December 1992.

35. K. G. Chapman and P. F. Winter, Electronic Identification and Signatures: A Response. *Pharm. Technol.* 16 (11): 36-46, 1992; and *Pharm. Technol. Int.*, pp. 20–30. January 1993.

Other Sources of Information, Guidelines, Controls, and Standards

Guidelines for the Documentation of Computer Software for Real-Time and Interactive Systems, 2nd Edition. Institution of

Electrical Engineers, Savoy Place, London, 1990. ISBN 0 86341 2335.

Software Quality Assurance: Model Procedures. Institution of Electrical Engineers, Savoy Place, London, 1990. NCC Blackwell Publishing Catalogue, NCC Blackwell, 108 Cowley Road, Oxford, OX4 1JF. UK.

The Recommended Reading List and Institutions listed in the TickIT Guide (Disc TickIT Office).

Guidelines for IT Management—National Computing Centre Manchester, M1 7ED, UK.

Designing Controls into Computerized Systems, J. Fitzgerald and Associates, 506 Barkentine Lane, Redwood City, CA 94065 USA, 1981. ISBN 0 9324100367.

PES—Programmable Electronic Systems in Safety Related Applications: 1. An Introductory Guide, ISBN 0 11 883913 6; 2. General Technical Guidelines, ISBN 0 11 883906 3. By the Health and Safety Executive. Published by HMSO, PO Box 276, London SW8 5DT, England.

Computerized Data Systems for Nonclinical Safety Assessment: Current Concepts and Quality Assurance. Published by Drug Information Association, Maple Glen, USA, September 1988.

Good Laboratory Practice Advisory Leaflet No. 1, *The Application of GLP Principles to Computer Systems.* UK GLP compliance programme, Department of Health, London, 1989.

Principles of Computer Use in a Regulated Pharmaceutical Industry. (memorandum/conclusions) EOQC, Berne, 1989. ISBN 3905538-03-2.

U.S. Environmental Protection Agency, *Good Automated Laboratory Practices* (Draft): Recommendations for Ensuring Data Integrity in Automated Laboratory Operations—with Implementation Guidance, December 1990.

Index

Center for Biologics Evaluation &
  Research (CBER), 276
Center for Drug Evaluation & Research
  (CDER), 276
certificate of analysis, 98, 129
certification, 260–263. *See also* validation
CFR. *See Code of Federal Regulations*
CGMPs, 24–27, 47, 51, 56, 203, 276
challenge testing, 259
change control
  data, 15, 21, 53
  documents for 68–71, 151–152
  for logic controllers, 257
  protocol for, 66, 101, 185, 202
  software, 183
    bug fixes vs. planned changes, 146
    in SDLC, 245, 251
    inspections and, 267
    problems in, 2
    procedures for, 189, 244
    SOPs for, 16, 177 (*see also* SOPs)
  system, 13, 74, 239, 264, 269, 280
    as best practice, 246
    documentation of, 49, 73, 253
    in integrated systems, 232
    in SDLC, 245
    inspections and, 199, 237
    procedures for, 7, 120, 213, 290,
      303, 305
    protocol for, 202
    responsibilities for, 7
    SOPs for, 16, 117
Chapman, K., 3, 10, 33, 72, 89, 90, 91, 198,
  214, 218, 219, 265, 293, 308, 309, 310
CIM, 60, 73, 74, 90, 88, 276
Clark, A. S., 308
clinical research associate (CRA), 161. *See
  also* CRA
code
  modification of, 255
  object, 282, 283
  review of, 133
  source (*see* source code)
Code of Federal Regulations (CFR), 22, 32,
  198, 276, 308
Commercial Off-the-Shelf (COTS) software, 83, 276, 280
Commission of the European
  Communities (CEC), 276
Committee on Proprietary Medicinal
  Products (CPMP) (UK), 19, 157,
  276. *See also* CPMP

common sense, 280
completion report, 68
Compliance Policy Guides (CPGs). *See* CPGs
computer assisted design (CAD), 275
computer assisted manufacturing (CAM), 275
computer-assisted new drug application.
  See CANDA
computer assisted software engineering
  (CASE), 275. *See also* CASE
computer disasters, 1–2
computer integrated manufacturing
  (CIM), 276. *See also* CIM
Computer Systems Validation Committee
  (CSVC) of U.S. PMA, 72, 90, 200,
  203, 276, 294
  elements of computerized system, 3
  expert systems, 88
  life cycle approach to validation, 26, 206
computerized system, 280
  building quality into, 4–5, 23
  inspector concerns of, 234–238
  people and procedures, 3–4, 9
  SOPs for (*see* SOPs)
  validation of, 79–80 (*see also* validation)
Comstock, T., 270
concurrent process validation, 87, 280
configurable software, 65
configuration management
  as best practice, 246
  certification and, 251
  data for, 53, 239
  for older systems, 255, 256
  in SDLC, 245
  inspection and, 237, 267
  need for, 3
  procedures for, 253
  QMS and, 251, 269
  SOPs for, 239
configured application, 113, 114, 209,
  253–254, 260
controlled process, 5
controlling system, 5, 126
corrective action, 30, 55, 235, 299
COTS, 83, 276
CPGs, 24–27, 32, 33, 90, 198, 219, 308
CPMP, 19, 31, 32, 162, 176, 276
CRA, 161, 170, 172
CRF, 20, 161, 275
  corrections to, 21, 174
  management system. 162, 163, 164, 166
  documentation of 169–170,
    171–172